# CLASSICAL HATHA YOGA

**84 classical Asanas and their variations**

**Yogacharyia Jnandev,**
Founder and Director
of Yoga Satsanga Ashram, Wales

© 2016 Yoga Satsanga Ashram,  Yogachariya Jnandev
design Vincenzo Schiraldi
illustrations Leonardo Mincuzzi

First Published June 2016
Published by Design Marque

Printed in Great Britain by
www.designmarque.co.uk

ISBN 978-0-9927841-5-7

This work on Classical Yoga Asanas is dedicated to my Parents for all their blessings, guidance, love and support throughout my life and yoga sadhana.

I believe in divine energy in the form of Guru the divine teacher who leads us from darkness to light. This work is a compilation of classical yoga asanas I have learned from various yoga masters and scriptures.

My first sincere gratitude and Pranams to Dr Swami Gitananda Giri Ji Guru Maharajaji for all the teaching and blessings on me through Ammaji Meenakshi Devi Bhavanani and Dr Ananda Balayogi Bhavanani. I would have never made this journey all this far without their guidance and blessings. I will truly recommend to all the one's who sincerely desire to learn yoga to learn under guidance of these true yoga masters at Ananda Ashram, Pondicherry.
*Visit www.icyer.com for more details.*

My sincere dedication and gratitude to great Yogi of Himalayas-Balendu Giriji, a great master teaching yoga in many schools in Jaipur, who guided me on Hatha-yoga teaching skills to children and teenagers.

Next I would like to offer my respect and gratitude to yoga master Mahavira Nathji of Natha tradition who provided me a safe place for my yoga sadhana and nurtured my soul with his blessings and divine love.

These above are just a few of the great masters who have blessed me with their yogic wisdom, although I am still grateful to many others who are not mentioned here.

My sincere thanks to Annapurna Helen (founder of Womankind Yoga and a catalyst motivator in healthy vegan food) for proof reading and editing work. She managed to find some time along with her busy schedule of yoga teachings, cooking and promoting vegan cooking, writing vegan blogs along with nurturing and growing her family with her husband and little Yolo. Also huge thanks to Sasha Kocho-Williams who did part of the very first edit.

I am grateful to Vincenzo for his design work and to Leonardo for amazing illustration work.

I am truly grateful to my three little young divine souls, Siddha, Mahadev and Krishna for their love and presence.

I am also grateful to Yogacharini Deepika my Dharma-Patni, or divine wife for all her support in my Sadhana and yoga work. Without her support I would have never been able to be where I am.

**Yogachariya Jnandev** (Surender Kumar Saini)
Founder and Director of Yoga Satsanga Ashram, Wales, UK.
M.Sc. Preksha Meditation and Yoga from Jain Vishwa Bharati, Ladnun, India.
6 months Residential Advance Teacher Training, from ICYER, Ananda Ashram, India.

Yogachariya Jnandev (Surender Saini) and Yogacharini Deepika (Sally Saini) are an integral part of my Gitananda Yoga family worldwide and I am so proud of the way they have been able to develop through hard work the Yoga Satsanga Ashram in Carmarthenshire, Wales. Having visited their Ashram, I can vouch for the beautiful spiritual ambience that can be felt there and it is a joy to teach in such a Yogic atmosphere.

This book focusing on Asana, the third limb of Maharishi Patanjali's Ashtanga Yoga, especaiily in the context of Hatha Yoga is indeed a labour of love and passion. Each and every one of the 84 asanas highlighted has been discussed with dedication and skill that will enable the reader to go deeper in their own Hatha Yoga Sadhana. Many of the variations ( Paravritti) on the different postures have also been detailed thus enabling the sincere seeker to realise that Yoga Sadhana is not static but is dynamic and ever changing as we grow and evolve on our spiritual journey towards Kaivalya (liberation).

A special word of appreciation for the artist who has so beautifully brought out the nuances of each and every posture and to the team that has done the editing work in the sense of true Karma Yoga Seva. May the Guru Parampara continue to bless Yogachariya Jnandev, Yogacharini Deepika and their family as well as the Yoga family of the Ashram with success in their Yoga Sadhana.

May we all grow and glow in spirit through the life of Yoga, enabling each and every one to manifest their inherent divinity with joy, health and wellness.

Om Hari Om tat Sat Om.

**Yogacharya Dr Ananda Balayogi Bhavanani**
Chairman: ICYER at Ananda Ashram, Pondicherry

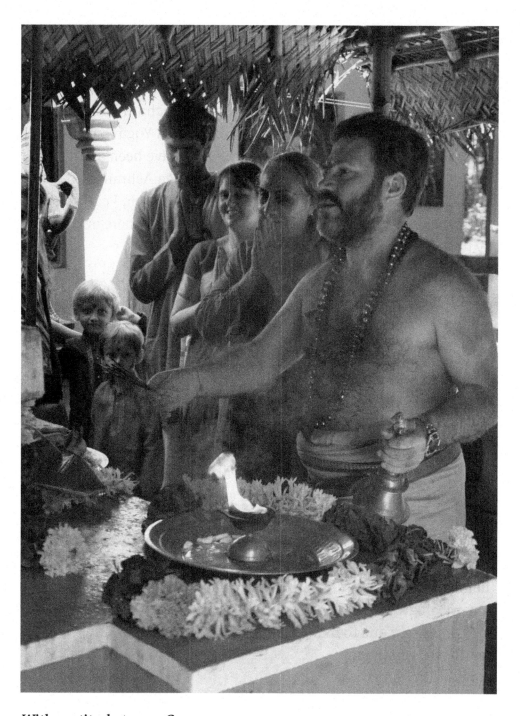

*With gratitude to our Gurus.*
In picture Jnandev and Deepika at Swami Gitananda Giri's Samadhi
in Kambaliswami Madam standing with Dr Ananda and Ammaji.

# CONTENT

## INTRODUCTION

## CHAPTER 1

### SURYANAMASKAR

## CHAPTER 2

### STANDING POSTURES

## CHAPTER 3

### ASANA PRACTICES AND SEQUENCES FROM VAJRASANA

## CHAPTER 4

### ASANA PRACTICES AND SEQUENCES FROM UTTANASANA (LEGS OUTSTRETCHED)

## CHAPTER 5
### ASANA PRACTICES AND SEQUENCES FROM CROSS LEGGED

## CHAPTER 6
### SEATED TWISTS

## CHAPTER 7
### ASANA PRACTICES AND SEQUENCES FROM FOUR FOOTED

## CHAPTER 8
### ASANA PRACTICES AND SEQUENCES FROM FACE PRONE

## CHAPTER 9
### INVERTED POSTURES

**CHAPTER 10**

**HAND OR ARM BALANCING POSTURES**

**CHAPTER 11**

**ASANA PRACTICES AND SEQUENCES FROM LYING ON SIDE**

**CHAPTER 12**

**ASANA PRACTICES AND SEQUENCES FROM SHAVASANA (SUPINE)**

## CHAPTER 13
### CLASSICAL SEATED POSTURES FOR MEDITATION

## YOGA: A PATH TO EVOLUTION AND LIBERATION

Yoga in its true meaning means union or oneness. Nowadays most people understand yoga as synonym of Asana/posture, and kriya/movement. The word yoga is a Sanskrita term derived from root 'yuj', which means adding, joining or uniting. Yoga means union with the self with the supreme self, or union of self with divine self.

Maharishi Patanjali explains Yoga as a path and goal. In the first sutra he describes yoga as discipline (atha-yoga-anushasanam: here is the discipline of yoga). Yoga includes kriyas and prakriyas, tools in forms of practices and their applications to grow physically, mentally, emotionally and spiritually. In verse 2 and 3 Patanjali explains yoga as stillness or quietness of mind and the absorption of mind in to Self itself. From verse 4 he describes that if not aware to our true self, our mind or chitta is busy in its own whirlpools. Here as a path, yoga provides us tools to clear, cleanse, unwind and unlearn all these whirlpools, ideas, concepts and experiences leading us into these whirlpools of mind, feelings, and emotions.

Swamiji Dr Gitananda Giriji mentions that, "Yoga is mother of all the sciences. Yoga is scientific, applicable and universal". Sciences are based on experiment and proof. Yoga has all the tools for health and well being, evolution and liberation. The Sadhaka needs to learn and follow all the practices, kriyas and prakriyas, asana and pranayama and experience the truth. Its also proved and experimented and experienced by thousands of Yoga Masters and Gurus, Rishis and Maharishis.

In Bhagavata Gita Lord Krishna describes yoga as follows: "Yoga is skill in action; Yoga is equanimity; Yoga is union; Yoga is devotion;

Yoga is meditation or one-pointed concentration."
All these definitions of yoga clearly describe yoga as skilful, mindful, harmonic, holistic living. Yogic living is evolutionary path to empower the self and enable one to experience and become one with the divine.

*Samkhya Yoga* describes yoga as a path of freeing the Purusha (Self) from all the gross elements and attributes and leading it in union or oneness with the Parmatman (Supreme Self). This whole universe, living and non-living aspects are composed of elements or bhutas or the evolutes of Cosmic energy or Divine self. Our true self is covered with our ego, i-ness, karma, whirlpools and states of mind, our memories, experiences and desires. Following yoga practices, yamas and niyamas and other aspects helps us to clear this covering from our soul, so it can shine freely and illuminate its light again.

Yoga has many paths and approaches, tools and applications, kriyas and prakriyas, moral restrains and observations, behavioural or habitual mental correctional approach through its wisdom and realisations. Yoga is holistic living, taking responsibility of our behaviour, actions and reactions, choices and decisions we make. Swamiji Gitananda states that "worldly and material people are **living to learn** whilst a **yogi learns how to live.**"

The Path of Evolution and Spiritualism is responsible and sensible living. This step by step approach or path of Raja Yoga has the following eight limbs or steps:

PANCHA YAMAS *Ahimsha* (non-harm), *Satya* (truthfulness), *Asteya* (non-stealing), *Brahmachariya* (continence), and *Aparigraha* (non- greed). Yamas deals with our moral and ethical behavior to refine our animal behavior patterns. Yamas can also be seen as how to fulfill our biological needs and desires. *Ahimsa* or non-violence, means abstaining from any violent activity on physical, mental, emotional and spiritual levels. We need to master yamas universally towards ourselves and other material and non-material aspects. The second Yama is *Satya* or truth, means abstaining lies, dishonesty, and manipulation of reality. The third Yama is *Asteya* or non-stealing means abstaining from stealing, or taking things that don't belong to us and not taking anything for granted. The fourth Yama is *Brahmchariya*, means abstaining from breaking the laws of nature and energy. Many translate this as sexual abstinance, as yoga is also path for householders and hence it should be translated as sexual discipline and channeling our energy into higher realizations and truth seeking instead of sensual pleasures. *Aparigraha* is the fifth and last of the Yamas, which means non-greed or detachment. Being free from accumulating things we don't need, letting go and freeing from clinging to material and non-material aspects.

PANCHA NIYAMA *Shaucha* (cleanliness), *Santosha* (contentment), *Tapas* (mortification), *Swadhyaya* (self-study), and *Isvara-pranidhana* (self-surrender to God) are the five Niyamas.

Niyamas are practices we all need to follow to achieve success in our goal. First Niyama is *Shaucha*, which means cleansing or hygiene. Keeping our body, mind, emotions clean and free from negativity. It also includes the cleanliness of our surroundings and environment. *Samtosha* is second Niyama means contentment or self-satisfaction. Being contented in outcomes or fruits of everything we do. This can also be seen as non-judgemental living. The next three Niyamas are also classified as Kriya Yoga and described in itself are enough to lead us to liberation or enlightenment. *Tapas*, the third Niyama means austerity or practice. Following and practicing our yoga daily with sincerity, regularity, faith and devotion. The fourth Niyama is *Swadhyaya* means intro-inspection or self study. Being aware to our body, mind and emotions is the first step towards *Swadhyaya*, which gradually can lead us to awareness of awareness itself. The fifth Niyama is *Isvara-Pranidhana*, which means surrendering to the divine. Swamiji Dr Gitananda Giriji translates it as seeing life and life events as divine blessing (isvara-prashadhanam).

**ASANA** Asana is the third limb of Raja Yoga, which means a seat, state or being, or throne. Patanjali describes asana as "sthiram sukham asanam" which means a "steady, stable, pleasant posture is Asana." Asana or posture is for achieving a healthy body and healthy mind so one can be comfortable in one position or asana for meditation and other higher practices. Various scriptures describe various number of postures like 84, 32 and out of them four meditation postures are the most important. These are *Sukhasana, Vajrasana, Padmasana* and *Siddhasana*. Hatha-Yoga-Pradipika, Gheranda Samhita and Yajnavalkya are some of the texts have great detail on Asana and Mudras. Asana is to refine, awaken and channel or gross energies to subtle energies.

**PRANAYAMA** Pranayama, controlling the vital forces of the body and mind is the forth limb of Raja Yoga. Pranayama is derived from Prana and Ayama. Prana means purest and subtlest forms of cosmic energy. It is all pervading, eternal and ever existing. Ayama means extension or lengthening. Breath is used as a tool to control, refine and channel our Prana. Pranayama is for cleansing our mind, nervous system, mental and emotional bodies and gradually refining gross prana or forces to subtle prana or life force or eternal cosmic energy. The Hatha-Yoga Pradipika describes eight classical Pranayamas. These are *Suriya and Chandra Nari, Bhastrika, Kapalbhati, Anuloma Viloma, Nari Sodhana, Bhramari, Kaki, Shitali and Shitakari* Pranayama. In the Gitananda tradition Swamiji used to teach around 120 Pranayamas.

**PRATYAHARA** Pratyahara, sensory withdrawal or introversion of mind and senses. This fifth limb of Raja Yoga deals with training our senses, mind and their fields of actions or attributes. We all are familiar with the five sense organs: eyes, nose, ears, tongue and skin. These are interactive bridges between our external and internal environment and help us to know what is going on around. Yoga describes 13 sense organs all together. The next five are known as *Karmendriyas* or instruments of action, or locomotive sense organs. These are the feet, the hands, excretion, reproduction and speech. The other three sense organs or instruments are mind, buddhi (or intellect) and ego. As in Pranayama we refine our energies, which is followed by *Pratyahara* as withdrawl and introversion of the subtle energies. This is also training our mind and senses to be able to focus inward to our vital energies and true self.

DHARANA Dharana, or concentration is the sixth limb. Patanjali mentions that Dharana or concentration is ability of mind. This limb includes a set of visualisations or practices to train our mind and engage or focus it on one point. This includes external and internal or conceptual visualisations and contemplations gradually leading us to realizing who we really are. *Kashmira Bhairava Tantra* deals in detail on more than 110 techniques of concentration.

In Bhagavat Gita Lord Krishna describes one of the most beautiful dharana or concentration. He says: "Choose a comfortable seat and posture with an erect spine. Gaze your mind on the tip of the nose and watch your inhaling and exhaling breath." Arjuna explains that every time he tries to do it, there seems to be more thoughts and whirlpools disturbing him. Krishna says: "If your mind wanders away 1000 times bring it back to your breath 1001 times! One day you will master your mind and concentration."

DHYANA Dhyana, or meditation is the seventh limb. Meditation is a state of being or mind-fullness when the practitioner is completely absorbed or becomes one with the point of focus or concentration.

*Ammaji Meenakshi Devi* describes concentration or dharana as "focusing more and more on less and less". Dhyana or meditation is not something you practice, it is a state of single-pointed mind we achieve. Yoga provides tools to achieve this state of realization or union.

**SAMADHI** Samadhi, or super-consciousness. Samadhi is the highest state of meditation or absorption of self in Self where that 'I' or ego doesn't exist anymore and the self becomes one with the higher self. This state is known as liberation, enlightenment, union, self-realization, etc.

## HATHA YOGA LEADS TO RAJA YOGA

Hatha Yoga is mainly known for its Shat-Karmas (six cleansing practices), Asana or posture, Mudra (seals of energy or gestures), Pranayama (breath and vital energy cleansing work), and some concentration techniques. Two widely known scriptures of Hatha Yoga are the *Hatha-Yoga-Pradipika* and *Gheranda Samhita*. In both the scriptures the masters of yoga explain that this part of yoga is to master our body, mind and energy to become eligible for Raja-Yoga.

If we are suffering aches and pain, injuries, health issues, mental and emotional clutter, how can we sit quietly and comfortably? We also carry all the memories and experiences in our vertebral or spinal memory which causes or helps in 'Fight or Flight' responses. Some of the traumatic memories, karmic bondages or impressions, emotionally suppressed or disturbed memories constantly keep arousing and affecting our body and mind. Simply what ever goes in our mind echoes or manifests in our body. If you are going through mentally disturbing memories, your muscles, heart, breathing, stomach and other systems are disturbed too, and vice-versa. Hatha or physical practices were designed by great Yogis and Masters to gain a healthy body, clean mind, harmonised breath and proper flow of vital energies throughout our Pancha-Koshas.

The Sanskrita term Hatha is derived from HA and THA. HA means solar, masculine, or pranic energy vibrating or flowing through the right side of our body. THA means lunar, feminine, or apanic energy flowing or vibrating through the left side of our body. Imbalance between the right and left, solar and lunar or masculine and feminine energy causes disturbed homeostasis of our body system and mental activities. With the modern Anatomy and Physiology perspective it can be seen in the form of autonomic nervous system and endocrine or hormonal imbalance. Hatha Yoga has the mean to establish homeostasis or balance of our body, mind and emotions to regain health, well-being and happiness.

Hatha also means with force or forcefully. Rishi Matsendra says: "Press your limbs against each other and it will lead you to health and well being." He followed his meditation in the Matsendrasana, which is a deep twist of spine and all the abdominal and pelvic organs are pressing against each other. All its variations are being used in curing and managing sugar problems, diabetes, heart troubles and digestive issues. Most Hatha Yoga practices are vigorous and intense and hence one should learn and practice them under guidance of a trained Hatha Yoga Master as it says in *Hatha-Yoga Pradipika* and *Gheranda Samhita*

## ASANA: THE THIRD LIMB OF ASHTANGA YOGA

Asana in modern yoga has become a synonym for Yoga. Most yoga followers are practising kriyas in the form of *Suriya-namaskar* or vinyasa and asana as a physical workout for many benefits like keeping fit, gaining flexibility, feeling good, being strong, looking attractive and enhancing vital energy. There is nothing wrong in that as we all need a healthy and strong body to begin. Swami Vivekananda states that, "all our immoral behaviour problems are rooted in weakness." To be free or to walk on a path to freedom and joy, we need to be very strong and healthy.

The word Asana in Sanskrita is derived from the Sanskrit root 'Aas' which means existence or state of existence. Asan is a Sanskrita term which means 'SEAT'. In Sanaskrita, Asana is also used in various contexts which gives a more holistic understanding of Asana. Asana means Yoni or form of birth. Asana means state of being. Asana also means throne. In general conversation some one might say who holds Asana in your family, community or country. This means: who leads them. Asana is also represented as honouring or respecting someone, like offering Asana or seat to a guest.

In *Shiva Samhita, Hatha Yoga Pradipika, Gheranda Samhita* and other scriptures there is mention of 8,400,000 Asanas, which means form of births or life, YONI. We all have to go through each and every life form to learn and experience to grow. Out of those they say only 84 are important. Out of those 84 only 32 are most important and out of those, 4 sitting postures are essential ones. To be successful in pranayama and meditation one needs to master one of them.

Classically in Yoga, Asana means the highest state of your individual being. Comfortable seat with positive image, idea, perception and experience of oneself is Asana. In each and every Yoga Asana or posture we follow through that higher or divine image of SELF and meditate in what we are doing or how we are holding.

Asana is also how we hold ourselves not only during practising your physical yoga but also in your day to day life. Some one with upright, comfortable and positive posture, with shoulders open, erect spine, chin up and a positive facial expression itself is attractive and elegant to everyone. We feel good, our self esteem is great, will power is high when we hold a good posture. In classical or Raja Yoga, Asana is a state of self-awareness in wich we hold our body, mind and senses together.

According to Patanjali there are three steps to Asana. First is taking the position. The second is being aware to your position and the third is letting go of effort and relaxing to be comfortable. He describes Asana as 'sthiram sukham asanam 2.46' this means a 'STEADY, COMFORTABLE BODY POSTURE'.

He follows in the next verse and explains that with effort we need to let go the tension, stress and discomfort and allow the mind to focus on SELF, or infinite divine energy (prayatna shaithilya ananta samapattibhyam, 2.47). Once you master the perfect posture or Asana, you become free from pain and suffering caused from duality or opposites like heat and cold, good and bad or pain and pleasure (tatah dvandva anabhighata, 2.48).

According to Patanjali and Hatha Yoga traditions practice of Asana and kriya should be slow, steady, and effortless with full awareness or attention. Our breath and mind should be merged with our practice. There should not be vigorous force, jerks and strains in your Hatha Yoga practice.

All our fast, vigorous, speedy movements and reactions are

controlled by our spinal or vertebral memory. While all our conscious actions, slow and rhythmic movements with breathing, mindful holding of limbs in various positions is controlled by our cerebral cortex which is the higher evolved part of the brain compared to the vertebral brain. This is why naturally you will feel more consciously empowered when you practice Hatha-Yoga slowly, in rhythm with breath.

So in true meaning Asana is taking and holding a pose in slow, controlled rhythmic movement. This should be followed with holding and maintaining the pose with steadiness, comfort and ease. Finally, releasing or letting go of the effort and focusing on SELF are the keys of Asana.

This approach of sadhana results in mastering our body and mind, their movements as well as functions, and their effects or responses on each other. This is a precondition of Pranayama and Dharana. Our body and mind naturally like to be relaxed and comfortable. We have this built in system of homeostasis where our body, systems, muscles and cells like to come to their normality. Hatha Yoga is an approach to retrain our body to be able to come back to normality or natural state of health and well being.

According to Hatha Yoga Pradipika, "One can achieve Sound Health, Stability, Lightness of Body and Mind through mastering Asana".

The Gheranda Samhita describes the benefit of Asana as follows, "Perfecting the Stability of Body and Mind is the result of Asana".

Some of the commonly seen benefits of Asana are increased efficiency, stamina, better immunity, quiet & calm mind, better control on emotions, positive attitude, better self belief and confidence.

Asanas can be classified in following categories:

**MEDITATIVE ASANAS** Postures used for meditation and quiet sitting. Some of them are *Padma-asana* (Lotus), *Siddha-asana* (Perfect), *Swastika-asana* ( Auspicious), *Vajra-asana* (thunderbolt).

**ASANAS FOR IMPROVING HEALTH** These postures help to improve our health and well being in general. Some of them are *Matsyendra-asana* (spinal twist), *Sarvanga-asana* (shoulder stand).

**RELAXING ASANAS** *Shava-asana* (corpse) and *Makara-asana* (crocodile), *Suriya Nari* and *Chandra Nari Asana* are a few of the relaxing Asanas.

We can also classify the Asanas from the position we start them as follows:

**SUPINE POSITION** Lying on the back in *Shava-asana*, like *Eka-Pada-Uttana-Asana* (single leg lift), *Hala-asana* (plough), *Chakra-asana* (wheel), *Setu-Asana* (bridge) etc.

**FACE PRONE POSITION** Asanas in lying on the front like *Bhujanga-asana* (cobra), *Shalabha-asana* (locust ), *Dhanura-asana* (Bow), etc.

**SEATED POSITION** Asanas in seated positions like *Padma-asana* (lotus) *Matsyendra-asana* (spinal twist), *Paschimottana-asana* (forward stretch), *Vajra-asana* (thunderbolt), etc.

**STANDING POSITION** Asanas performed from standing position like *Trikona-asana* (triangle), *Veera-asana* (warrior pose), *Vriksha-asana* (tree pose) etc.

# GENERAL BENEFITS OF HATHA YOGA OR ASANA PRACTICE

There are so many benefits of Yoga to mention. Plenty follow yoga for some basic benefits like weight loss, flexibility, suppleness, pain relieve, stress release, mental peace, emotional stability, physical strength, better sleep, healthy posture, etc. Here are some holistic benefits of Hatha Yoga practice.

**PHYSICAL STRENGTH** Regular practice of hatha-yoga or posture work will strengthen the body. It helps strengthen muscles, joints, bones and inner organs. Hatha Yoga practice improves blood and energy circulation.

**FLEXIBILITY, MOBILITY AND COORDINATION** Stiffness caused by poor diet, unhealthy life style, and lack of proper exercise gradually results in tensed muscles, stiff joints, lack of flexibility, lack of stability or steadiness, coordination of limbs and body parts. Yoga can help in preventing or curing the stiffness, bring flexibility, mobility and coordination. Teaching plenty of kriya work with breath and sound will also help yoga practitioners to enjoy and find coordination. Yoga will benefit in improving flexibility, mobility, and healthy muscles and joints.

**ENDURANCE AND CAPACITY** We all need to have endurance, the capacity to deal with physical, mental and emotional strains and the pressures we have to go through. Yoga will help prepare our muscular and organ strength as well as their capacity to deal with all the challenges. Yoga balances the hormones and autonomic nervous system.

**STABILITY AND CONCENTRATION** In our day-to-day tasks it is very important to be focused and stable in tasks we are engaged in. If we are unstable or unable to focus, it results in a struggle in day-to-day tasks and learning activities. This can gradually build the pressure and cause more serious mental and emotional problems. Regular Asana and pranayama practice will help improve stability and concentration and hence yoga can be very helpful in preventing many mental and emotional problems too.

**MENTAL AND EMOTIONAL BALANCE** All the pressure and competition in our modern life style causes mental and emotional imbalance and it disturbs our day-to-day balance and behaviour. Yoga also prepares and balances mental and emotional behaviours through strengthening and empowering our body, mind and soul.

**WILL POWER, SELF CONFIDENCE AND ENTHUSIASM** As yoga offers a wide range of practices at each and every level' hence every one can appreciate and enjoy as well as be encouraged and motivated further more to gradually help them improve their control and mastery of their body. This improves self-confidence, will power and enthusiasm for doing things and accepting challenges.

**DISCIPLINE** In yoga it is said that discipline is the only path to freedom and success. Weaknesses, lack of stability, fear, etc. cause the irritation, anger and agitation, which results in lack of discipline. Yoga empowers the self, removes all the weaknesses and fear.

**MORAL AND ETHICAL VALUES** Lots of behaviour problems are rooted in a weak body. If we want to have a healthy and ethical society, the first key element will be a healthy and strong physique. Swamiji Dr Gitananda Giriji mentions that yoga and evolution is the path for strong and brave people. This also means that only strong people can follow the holistic life style. Moral and ethical values are one of the key factors for improving our life and establishing peace around us. Hatha Yoga leads into Raja Yoga which provides all the tools at this level.

**SELF RESPECT AND CARING** We also need to learn to respect and care for ourselves as well as others. Hatha Yoga and posture work also helps us to know ourselves better. This helps us to appreciate and respect what we do, what we have and what we achieve.

**HOLISTIC HEALTH AND WELL-BEING** Holistic well being on a physical, mental, emotional, social and spiritual level can be empowered through Hatha Yoga. Hatha Yoga including Asana, Pranayama, Mudra and Meditation is a holistic package of over-all health and well-being.

## ASANA IN HATHA YOGA SCRIPTURES

If we begin with Maharishi Patanjali, he simply means Asana as a comfortable seat for meditation. And he puts Asana as the third limb in Ashtanga Yoga and explains all about Asana in three verses all together. In ancient holistic and authentic yoga, physical attachment was seen as one of the causes of suffering and yoga was the path to be free from bodily attachment.

The Maitrayai Upanishad explains as follows "Venerable, in this ill-smelling, unsubstantial body, which is nothing but a conglomerate of bone, skin, muscle, marrow, flesh, semen/eggs, blood, mucus, tears, rheum, feces, urine, wind, bile, and phlegm—what good is the enjoyment of desires? In this body, which is afflicted with desire, anger, greed, delusion, fear, despondency, envy, separation from the desirable, union with the undesirable, hunger, thirst, senility, death, disease, sorrow, and the like—what good is the enjoyment of desires?"

All those ancient Yoga Masters, Rishis and Swamijis believed that to become free from the cycle of birth, death and re-birth we must first become free of attachment to our physical bodies. It was later between the 4th and 6th Century Tantra explored the non-dualistic aspect of our spirit, divine and its creation. If the cosmic or consciousness is all pervading then body is divine too as it is also manifestation of Spirit.

So in Tantra, Georg Feuerstein explains as follows: "Instead of regarding the body as a meat tube doomed to fall prey to sickness and death, they viewed it as a dwelling place of the Divine and as the vehicle for accomplishing spiritual perfection."

Later on the Siddha yogis developed the Asanas or postures, Pranayama or breathing exercises, Mudras or energy seals and Shata Karmas or purification techniques of Hatha Yoga. Hatha Yoga is believed to have originated with Matsyendra Natha and Goraksha Natha in the ninth or tenth centuries in one of the greatest Hindu Monk and Yoga traditions. And it was kept secret. One needed to be Adhikari (eligible one) and prove it to the Guru to learn all these hatha Yoga techniques traditionally. Even after the texts were written later it clearly mentioned that the practices must be kept secret and learned from the Yoga Masters. Really most practices in scriptures are in codified forms.

Three Hatha Yoga texts are considered primary: the *Hatha Yoga Pradipika, Shiva Samhita, and Gheranda Samhita*. After these scriptures generally Asana was known as Hatha Yoga Practice.

According to scholars, the *Hatha Yoga Pradipika* was written in the fourteenth century; the *Shiva Samhita* may have been written in the late fifteenth or late seventeenth centuries and the *Gheranda Samhita* was written in the late seventeenth century. The *Gheranda Samhita* is the most detailed scripture on Asana. The *Hatha Yoga Pradipika* in a chapter, known as Asana, explains: "Being the first step or limb of Hatha Yoga, asana is described first. It should be practiced for attaining a steady posture, and a healthy and light body."

Then Svatmarama Suri the Hatha Yoga master names 15 postures. Eleven of them are *Svastikasana* (auspicious posture), *Gomukha-asana* (cow face posture), *Vira-asana* (hero posture), *Kurma-asana* (tortoise posture), *Kukkuta-asana* (cock posture), *Uttana kurma-asana* (intense tortoise posture), *Dhanura-asana* (bow posture), *Matsya-asana* (fish posture), *Paschimottana-asana* (back stretch posture), *Mayura-asana* (peacock posture), and *Sava-asana* (corpse posture). After mention of these eleven postures, he further says- "Shiva taught 84 asanas, and of these the four are essential ones." These are four seated postures: *Siddha-asana* (perfect posture), *Padma-asana* (lotus posture), *Simha-asana* (lion posture), and *Bhadra-asana* (fortunate posture).

The *Shiva Samhita* states as follows: "This temple of suffering and enjoyment, made up of flesh, bones, nerves, marrow, blood and intersected with blood vessels etc. is only for the sake of suffering of sorrow... This body, the abode of Brahma, and composed of fine elements and known as Brahmanda (the egg of Brahma or microcosm) has been made for the enjoyment of pleasure or suffering of pain."

The *Shiva Samhita* describes four: *Siddha-asana, Padma-asana, Ugra-asana,* and *Svastika-asana.* The *Shiva Samhita*, in the fourth chapter on Mudras, describes *Mahamudra*, or *Janusirsasana* as one more posture.

The *Gheranda Samhita* explains about Asana as follows: "There are 8,400,000's of Asanas described by Shiva. The postures are as many in number as there are numbers of species of living creatures in this universe. Among them 84 are the best; and among these 84, 32 have been found useful for mankind in this world."

Here is the list of 32 postures from *Gheranda Samhita*:
*Siddha-asana, Padma-asana, Badhrasana, Muktasana, Vajrasana, Svastikasana, Simhasana, Gomukhasana, Ardha-Virasana, Dhanurasana, Shavasan, Guptasana or Gupta Padmasana, Matsyasana, Matsyendrasana, Gorakshasana, Pashchimottanasana, Utkatasana, Sankatasana, Mayurasana, Kurmasana, Uttanakurmasana, Mandukasana, Uttanamandukasana, Vrikshasana, Garudasana, Vrishasana, Shalabhasana, Makarasana, Bhujangasana, Yogasana and Janusirsasana.*

# DRISTI OR GAZING POINT IN ASANAS

In ancient Hatha Yoga traditions each asana is associated with Dristi. Dristi means gazing, or fixed eye sight. Dristi is to prepare and practice Pratyahara or fifth limb and Dharana or concentration, the sixth limb of Raja Yoga.

**ANGUSTHA-MADHYE** Angushtha means thumb and Madhya means in the middle. So in *Angustha-Madhye dristi* you focus your gaze and mind on the middle of thumb. In *Vira-Bhadra Asana, Namaskar Mudra, Agra Namaskar Mudra* are some of the examples where you use this dristi.

**BHRU-MADHYE** Bhru means eyebrows and madhye means in the middle. In this dristi one gazes between the eyebrows at the third eye. This stimulates olfactory and optic nerves and gradually awakens and balances the autonomic nervous system and central nervous system. This also relieves and relaxes cranial nerves and helps improve concentration and helps awakening the third eye or Ajna chakra. *Siddhasana, Padmasana, Vajrasana, Meru Asana* are few examples where yogis describe to practice *Bhru-madhye dristi.*

**NASAGRE DRISTI** Nasa-agre, where Nasa means nose and agre means front or tip. So Nasagre means the tip of the nose. This is to strengthen eye muscles and concentrations. In Bhagavat Gita, Lord Krishna explains on Dhyana or meditation with this dristi as follows: "Sit comfortably in a meditative posture, with erect spine and gaze on the tip of your nose. Now watch your in and out breath. This dristi is advised to use in any meditative pose".

**HASTAGRAHE DRISTI** Hasta means hand and grahe means taking. Hastagrahe means the middle of the palms. Like in *Uthita*

*Trikonasana* and *Konasana* are two examples where you can gaze your dristi at the middle of the palms.

**PARSHYA DRISTI** This means gazing at the right or left side like in *Parshva-Konasana*, and *Janu-sirsasana Provritti*.

**URDHYA DRISTI** Urdhya means above or rising it eyes gazing over to the sky or upward beyond the body like in *Anjali mudra*, and *Ustrasana*.

**NAMBHICHAKRE DRISTI** Nabhi means navel, and chakra means circle or center. So Nabhichakre Dristi means gazing at the navel center. *Navasana*, and *Meru Asana* are two example postures for this dristi.

**PADAYORAGRE DRISTI** Pada means feet and agre means front or tip, so Padayoragre means at the tip of the feet. *Paschimottanasana* and *Hasta-Pada-Asana* are the two best examples for this dristi.

# HATHA YOGA: THE SADHANA OF KALI YUGA

**AN ARTICLE BY OUR ESTEEMED TEACHERS:**

*Yogacharini Meenakshi Devi Bhavanani*
Director, ICYER at Ananda Ashram, Pondicherry, India.
*Yogacharya Dr Ananda Balayogi Bhavanani*
Chairman ICYER at Ananda Ashram, Pondicherry, India.

"YOGA" is an ancient Sanskrit word which, in only two syllables, encompasses the entire body of spiritual experiences and experiments of thousands of Realised Masters. These Masters have discovered the *Ultimate Reality*, *Sat*, and in their infinite compassion, carefully marked a path for others to follow. The *Upanishads* exclaim: "Lo! Ye who suffer know! A way has been found! A way out of all this darkness!" That way .... is Yoga!"

Yoga is as old as the Universe, for it is both the Path and the Goal. The Goal is realisation of the *Innate Nature of the Universe, the Highest Being: Atman, Purusha, Shiva, Devi, Sat...* whatever word we wish to use to describe its essence. In Sankhya and Yoga, that *Highest Being* is called *Purusha* – and the manifestation of That Spirit in the world of matter and senses is called *Prakriti*. It is through experiences in the *Prakriti*, or manifested world, that the *Jiva*, individual soul, returns to the *Paramatman*, or *Universal Soul*, Hence, *Purusha* and *Prakriti* are one and the same: *Purusha* is the Goal and *Prakriti*, the path to that Goal.

The word "*Yoga*" is often described as "*union*". It implies that the individual is united with the Universe, the personality with the Universality. The root of the word "*Yoga*" is the Sanskrit Bija "*Yuj*" which means "to join together." The English word '*yoke*' is directly derived from the Sanskrit "*Yuj*". In fact, the English word "*Union*" has a sound similar to *"Yuj"*. Perhaps one could more correctly say, Yoga is *"re-union"*. The *Upanishad* says: "That which was Onebecame the many." *Purusha* unfolded into the multi-splendrous material creation through *Prakriti*. The science of Yoga accelerates the "return of the many to the One", the re-union of *Purusha* and *Prakriti*, *Shivan* and *Shakti*, *Ram* and *Sita*. Thus, Yoga is both the Goal (*Purusha*) and the path to that Goal (*Prakriti*).

In this Cosmic Drama, Play, *Leela*, the sense of *Dwaitam*, the sense of separateness rose. From this *Dwaitam* (duality, two-ness) rose *Bhayam*, fear. The *Upanishad* says: "Where there are two, there is fear." This primordial fear rising from the sense of separateness is the root cause of all man's sufferings. That primordial fear can be destroyed when the Highest Sense of Oneness is once more achieved. The sages call this reunion, *Moksha, Samadhi, Kaivalya or Mukti*. This is the true goal of Yoga.

Mankind according to the Hindu world view degenerates physically, mentally and emotionally as the Wheel of Time revolves downward from Sat Yuga, through Treta Yuga, Dwapara Yuga and into the present age known as Kali Yuga. Kali Yuga is marked by the degeneration of human and social values: men are said to be "25% good and 75% evil". The description of this age in the scriptures is that families fall apart, the leaders are corrupt, institutions decay and men are no longer virtuous. The sages also advised that since in Kali Yuga, mankind is preoccupied with his body the best Sadhana is *Hatha Yoga,* or the Science of Achieving Higher Consciousness through disciplines of body and breath. Since *Hatha Yoga* has its origins in *Tantra*, the *Tantra* was also considered the *Sadhana of Kali Yuga.*

According to Yogamaharishi Dr Swami Gitananda Giri Guru Maharaj, founder of ICYER at Ananda Ashram, Pondicherry, India, the word "*Hatha*" is composed of two syllables: "HA" which refers to the solar, positive, warm, activating energies and "THA" which refers to the lunar, cooling, negative, inhibitive energies. "*Hatha Yoga*" thus becomes a method of creating a harmonious interaction or polarity between these two powerful, dialectically opposed primordial universal energies. The dominant right side of the body is harmonized with the more passive left side. The creative, intuitive, visionary right side of the bi-cameral brain is "yoked" harmoniously with the logical, rational, mathematically inclined left side of the brain. A polarized duality is transformed into a harmonious unity and the human personality becomes integrated. Then, real *Yoga* or Union occurs spontaneously. All this can be achieved by an aware, step-by-step, conscious, intelligent approach to *Asanas, Kriyas, Mudras, Bandhas, Pranayama* and *Jattis*, which are the technology of *Hatha Yoga*. Only when the being exists in a perfect Polarity of Prana – Apana, can the highest experience – Samadhi – occur.

## HATHA YOGA: A TOOL OF CONSCIOUS EVOLUTION.

Hatha Yoga is the perfect tool to help man evolve efficiently out of his animal tendencies into human qualities and then, to obtain transcendence into Divine realms of being. Yogamaharishi Dr. Swami Gitananda Giri taught his students the concept of "Four-Fold Awareness". One must, he said, first become aware of the body. The Second Awareness is awareness of emotions, senses and energy. The Third Awareness is awareness of mind. And the Fourth Awareness is of awareness itself". Good Hatha Yoga fosters deep awareness of the body inside-outside, right-side, left-side, to side, bottom side. The practices stimulate deep consciousness in every cell. This awareness "spills over" into an awareness of emotions, sensations, and energy, (prana flows). The awareness deepens into an awareness of the working of the mind, and how body, emotions, sensations and Prana are inseparably linked together. This deepening of consciousness enables the practitioner to direct the course of his own life activities, rather than be a victim of haphazard Karmic forces. Consciousness is the key to control and Hatha Yoga fosters consciousness. One becomes deeply aware of old reptilian and animal instincts lurking in the primordial sub-conscious. The various practices purify and exorcise these old animal / reptilian conditionings. Swamij Gitananda ji often explained this by saying: "All of the evolutionary history of life on this earth planet is contained in your brain. You have a reptilian brain and a mammalian brain, in common with those lower life forms and all their primordial instincts for survival: sexual drive, dominance, territoriality etc. are also active there. Then, you have the cerebral cortex, the human brain, which is no longer bound by instinct, but can make conscious choices. The problem facing man today is the lack of communication between this **"old, unconscious brain"** and the **"new conscious brain"**. **Hatha Yoga is the superb technology which enables man to bridge that gap**."

This is the reason why the ancient Rishis taught their disciples to put their bodies into positions resembling lower life forms like trees, mountains, insects, birds and animals. The *body remembers* those past incarnations *consciously when locked back into a form resembling those physical structures*. By becoming "*conscious of the unconscious*" the Jiva develops the perspective necessary to view with *Vairagya* (detachment) all the old animal and reptilian conditionings. This detached witnessing puts space between stimulus – response and one can choose consciously how one will respond to situations rather than react with the animal response of "flight or fight".

**HATHA YOGA AND ITS TEXTS**

In Vedic times the goal of the refined human was to seek Moksha, freedom from human birth and mergence in Cosmic Consciousness Asana meant a seated position or a seat. The word Asana is found in the *Bhagavad Gita*. In this sense it means simply "a seat", "a place to sit" or a seated position. The only physical instruction Lord Krishna gives Arjuna is "to sit straight, with head and neck erect". Indian Pandits date the *Bhagavad Gita* at least 5000 years ago. The next time the word "Asana" appear with significance is in the *Yoga Sutras* of Patanjali about 800 BCE. Patanjali simply says that Asana is the third of eight steps to liberation and is a body posture which is *sthiram sukham* (comfortable and steady). The original meaning of the word *Asana* could be derived from the root "*Asi*" which means "*to be*". Hence, *Asana* is a body position which enables the seeker to discover his true Being (God head) by remaining still and silent.

About 500 A.D. the emphasis of spirituality and Yoga started to shift more and more to physical practices and techniques in keeping with the materialistic, sensual, body-oriented nature of mankind in Kali Yuga. Certain "Yogic practices" evolved out of the *Atharva Veda* and the *Tantric* tradition which used the body itself as an instrument of *Sadhana*. Though these "techniques" were written down, they were written in a "coded language", making it impossible for the uninitiated to understand them. From about 500 A.D. to about 1500 A.D, several scriptures were recorded which are commonly known as the "Hatha Yoga Scriptures." These include the *Goraksasatakam*, the *Gheranda Samhita* and *Hatha Yoga Pradipika*. These three can be said to be the most prominent though many others exist.

This scripture was composed in 100 verses by the *Rishi Goraksha* who perhaps lived about 1500 years ago. Goraksha was a disciple of Matsyendra Nath, a wild mystic Tantric. Rishi Goraksha was a widely traveled Yogi with a towering personality who greatly influenced the masses of his day. He traveled the country challenging people to "breathe, breathe, and live". He is a representative of the Natha School and in his work, are many practical techniques of Yoga written down for the benefit of seekers. He preached the ideal of "*Samaradhya*", or the "sweetest and most perfect adjustment and harmony in one's life experience." Verse 4 defines the subject matter of Yoga: "Asanam pranasamyamah pratyaharoath dharana dhyanam samadhiretani yoganjgani bhavanti sat." "The six limbs of Yoga are Asana, Pranayama, Pratyahara, Dharana, Dhyanam and Samadhi". The entire text describes how these limbs may be achieved. Goraksha comes close to the Vedic ideal by emphasizing complete control of the physical organism and metal steadiness as the prelude to experiencing non-duality on the highest spiritual plane. He says there are 84 lakhs of Asanas. This idea is also found in THE SHIVA SAMHITA which says that the particular form of each living creature is an "Asana", as Lord Shiva holds still for a moment in his Cosmic Dance. Thus, there are 84 lakhs of species. Shiva has enumerated 84 important Asanas. Sage Goraksha says that of these, two Asanas are important, namely, *Siddhasana* and *Kamalasana*, which are both sitting meditative poses. Rishi Goraksha gives detailed information on the Chakras, or vortexes of spiritual energy located in the human energy field. He also teaches that there are thousands of Nadis, which serve as the pathways for Prana. Of these pathways, he says 72 are important.

The three most important Nadis are *Ida* (left side and deity is moon); *Pingala* (right side with deity as sun) and *Sushumna* (centre with deity as Agni or fire). He also describes the types of Prana, circulating in various parts of the human force field.

Rishi Goraksha also teaches of Kundalini, "She lies above the Kanda, folded eight times, always closing up by her mouth the entrance to the Brahmarandhra". "Kandordhava kundalisaktirsatadha kundalikrita brahmdrarmukham nityam mukhenavrtya tishtati. (G.S. 30) Rishi Goraksha also describes Pranayama practices, emphasizing *Puraka*, *Rechaka* and *Kumbhaka*. This is also dealt with in the system of concentration or Dharana taught by Rishi Goraksha which includes contemplation on the various Mandalas for the Pancha Maha Bhutas of earth, water, fire, air and ether. Samadhi or Cosmic Consciousness is also dealt with by the sage. He defines this highest spiritual state as: "When the Prana becomes stilled and the mind is absorbed, there result the identification of Jivatma and Paramatma which is called Samadhi". "Yada sanksiyate prano mausam ca vitiyate, tada a samarsaikatvam samadhirbhidhiyate" (G.S. 94). The measurements of the time duration needed for the state of Dharana to slip into Samadhi is also given in detail.

## THE GHERANDA SAMHITA

The basis of Indian spirituality is the negation of the *Ahamkara*, the ego, the sense of self, I-ness and mine-ness. Thus it is that for many of our greatest works of art in temples, sculptures, and scriptures, the author or creator's name is unknown. So it is with the GHERANDA SAMHITA. This self-abnegation of the Indian spiritual mind has made it very difficult for historians to accurately pinpoint time and place of both the various scriptures and the lives of the Masters. This scripture is in the form of a dialogue between *Gheranda*, the Preceptor, and *Chandakapali*, the disciple. Though it is a treatise of *Hatha Yoga*, it does not use the word

"*Hatha*". Instead, it calls the type of Yoga discussed in the treatise, "*Ghatastayoga*". This term is not found in any other text on Yoga. "*Ghata*" in this sense refers to the "*body*", and its literal meaning in Sanskrit also is "*a pot*". This suggests that the malleable "clay of the body" can be formed and fired by the practices of Yoga to make it a fit container to hold the "*waters of liberation*".

A beautiful statement by this Rishi occurs in G.S.1.4 "There are no fetters like those of illusion (*Maya*); No strength like that which comes from discipline (*Yoga*); there is no friend higher than knowledge (*Jnana*) and no greater enemy than egoism (*Ahamkara*). Whereas Yogamaharishi Patanjali calls Yoga as "*Ashtanga*", (Eight Limbs) and Rishi Goraksha calls Yoga as "*Shadanga*", (Six Limbs) Rishi Gheranda enunciates "*Saptayoga*" or "Seven Limbs" of Yoga. According to this Rishi the seven exercises for making the body fit for Divine Wisdom include: purificatory, strengthening, steadying, calming and those leading to lightness, perception and isolation. (Sudhanain dradhata caiva sthairyam dhairyam cal lagharam, pratyaksam ca nirilipatm ca ghatasya sapta sadhnam. G.S.1:9). Rishi Gheranda classifies the Yoga practices as:

1. Kriyas: Dhautis, Bastis, Neti, Trataka, Nauli, Kapalbhatis
2. Asanas
3. Mudras
4. Pratyahara
5. Pranayama
6. Dhyana
7. Samadhi.

Great emphasis is given to the purificatory practices which are quite elaborate. *Asanas* have been described in great detail in this work. Again we find the concept of 84 lakhs of Asanas enumerated by Lord Shiva. There are as many Asanas as there are creatures on earth. "Asanani samasthani yavante jivajantavah, caturasiti laksaru sivena kathithanica" (G.S.2.1). Among these, says the Rishi, eighty-four are best, and of those eighty-four, thirty-two have been found useful for mankind. The thirty-two Asanas recorded by Rishi Gheranda are: 1. *Siddam* (Perfect Posture); 2. *Padmam* (Lotus Posture); 3. *Bhadram* (Gentle Posture); 4. *Muktam* (Free Posture); 5. *Vajram* (Adamant Posture); 6. *Swastika* (Prosperous Posture); 7. *Sinham* (Lion Posture); 8. *Gomukha* (Cow-mouth Posture); 9.*Vira* (Heroic Posture); 10. *Dhanur* (Bow Posture); 11. *Mritam* (Corpse Posture) 12. *Guptam* (Hidden Posture); 13. *Matsyam* (Fish Posture); 14. *Matsendra*; 15. *Goraksha*; 16. *Paschimottana*; 17. *Utkatam* (Hazardous Posture); 18. *Sankatam* (Dangerous Posture); 19. *Mayuram* (Peacock Posture); 20. *Kukkutam* (Cock Posture); 21. *Kurma* (Tortoise Posture); 22. *Uttana Manduka*; 23. *Uttana Kurmakam*; 24. *Vriksha* (Tree Posture); 25. *Manduka* (Frog Posture); 26. *Garuda* (Eagle Posture); 27. *Vrisham* (Bull Posture); 28. *Salabha* (Locust Posture); 29. *Makara* (Dolphine Posture); 30. *Ushtram* (Camel Posture); 31. *Bhujangam* (Snake Posture); 32. *Yoga Mudra* (gesture of Yoga).

Twenty five Mudras are discussed, and afterward, Lord Shiva is quoted as telling Devi: "O Devi. I have told you all the Mudras. Their knowledge leads to adeptship. It should be kept secret with great care and should not be taught indiscriminately to everyone. This gives happiness to the Yogis". Again we see the idea that Yoga knowledge should be kept secret.

This great Rishi also discusses *Pratyahara* and *Pranayama* techniques laying emphasis first on the purification of the Nadis, asking: "Vayu cannot enter the Nadis so long as they are full of impurities. How then can Pranayama be accomplished? First, the Nadis should be purified".

Sage Gheranda also discusses *Dhyana* and *Samadhi* in detail. He divides *Dhyana* into three types: "Dhyana or meditation is of three kinds; gross, subtle and luminous. When a particular figure, such as one's Guru or Deity is contemplated, it is Sthula or gross; when Brahman or Prakriti is contemplated as a mass of light it is called Jyothi meditation; when Brahman as a Bindu (point) and Kundali force is contemplated, it is Sukshma or subtle meditation". (G.S. 6:1).

## HATHA YOGA PRADIPIKA

The *Hatha Yoga Pradipika* is of later authorship, perhaps written about 500 – 700 years ago. Even today, *Hatha Yoga Pradipika* is claimed to be the source book of instruction by many Yoga teachers. It was authored by Yogi Swatmarama Suri. It is divided into four Chapters. The first chapter is on *Asanas*; the Second Chapter is on *Pranayama*; the third chapter is on *Mudras* and the fourth chapter on *Samadhi*. Sage Swatmarama Suri in his second verse proclaims that "Swatmarama Yogin, having saluted his Lord and Guru, teaches the Hatha Vidya solely for the attainment of Raja Yoga. (Chapter I, V.2)" In 389 verses the sage gives fairly detailed instruction in Asanas, Pranayama, Mudras and means of attaining Samadhi. Sage Swatmarama Suri describes only fifteen Asanas, of which a few resemble those common in today's Hatha Yoga. He describes four of these Asanas, as the "best among postures". They are *Siddha Asana, Padma Asana, Simha Asana* and *Bhadra Asana* (Verse 33 Chapter One).

The Asanas described by Swatmarama Suri in Verse 19 through 32 of Chapter One are as follows: *Swastika Asana, Gomukhasana, Vira Asana, Kurma Asana, Kukkut Asana, Uttana Kurma, Dhanur Asana, Matsyendra Asana, Paschimmotana Asana, Mayura Asana and Shava Asana.* In Verse 33 of Chapter One he says: "The Asanas propounded by Lord Shiva are eighty-four in number. Of these I shall describe four which are the quintessence". In Verse 34 he continues: "These four are Siddha, Padma, Simha and Bhadra (Asanas) are most excellent. Of these four, the most comfortable, Siddha Asana, can always be assumed. "In the remaining verses of the first chapter, the Guru also discusses which foods are to be eaten. He recommends: "filling half the stomach with food, one quarter with water and leaving one fourth of the stomach free as an offering to Lord Shiva". (H.Y.P. Chapt, I, V.58).

In Chapter Two entitled PRANAYAMA the Shat Karmas or "Six Purificatory Acts" are described. They include *Dhauti, Vasti, Neti, Trataka, Nauli* and *Kapalabhati*. However, the Guru says in Verse 21. Chapter II: ".... One who is flabby and phlegmatic should first practise these six acts. Others who do not have these defects should not practise them". In Verse 44 of Chapter Two, he lists eight kinds of *Kumbhakas* (Pranayamas). "The different Kumbhakas are now described: There are eight Kumbhakas, namely Surya Bhedana, Ujjayi, Sitkari, Sitkali, Bhastrika, Bhramari, Murcha and Plavini".

In Verse 76 of Chapter II, he says: "One cannot obtain perfection in Raja Yoga without Hatha Yoga, nor perfection in Hatha Yoga without Raja Yoga, so both should be practised till perfection (in Raja Yoga) is obtained." In Chapter Three, Sage Swatmarama Suri describes the Mudras in Verses 6 and 7. "Maha Mudra, Maha Bandha, Maha Vedha, Khecari, Uddiyana, Mula Bandha, Jalandhara Bandha, Viparitakaranai, Vajroli and Shaktichalana, these are the ten Mudras. They destroy old age and death". He also gives instructions in arousal of Kundalini. Chapter Four is devoted to instructions in obtaining Samadhi. In Verse Five of Chapter Four, he says, "Samadhi is explained: As salt in water unites and dissolves with it, a likewise merging of mind and self is Samadhi". Verse 6. "When Prana is without any movement in Kumbhaka and the mind is absorbed in the Self, the state of harmony is called Samadhi".

Swatmarama Suri also mentions 72,000 *Nadis* and claims only *Sushumna Nadi* is of importance. He describes many methods of achieving the Samadhi state. He puts most emphasis on the use of *Nada*, or Inner Sound. He says in Verse 66, Chapter Four: "The primeval Lord Shiva has expounded one crore and a quarter of effective ways for the attainment of Laya (absorption) but we think that one thing, devotion to Nada, alone is the most important of all these ways".

Again in Verse 94, Chapter Four he says: "Nada is like the net which ensnares the deer (the mind) and it is also the hunter who slays the deer within (the mind)." He describes many aspects of Nada Yoga and also Samadhi. Swatmarama Suri concludes his work with Verse 114 of the Fourth Chapter, "As long as the Prana does not flow in the central way (through Sushumna) and enter the Brahmarandhra, as long as the semen does not become steady through restraint of breath, so long as the mind does not in meditation reflect the natural state (of the object contemplated upon, i.e. Brahman), so long as those who talk of spiritual knowledge indulge only in boastful and false prattle" (there is no success in Yoga).

In the HATHA YOGA PRADIPIKA, unlike other texts discussed thus far, much practical instruction is given in Asanas, Pranayama, Mudras and even in methods of attaining Samadhi. Yet, the instruction given is couched in difficult and deliberately obscure language. It is not a textbook on Yoga and Yoga practices could not be undertaken merely on the basis of studying the text. The references are far too obscure and too ambiguous. The Guru himself makes many references throughout the work, for the need for the practices to be kept secret. If he intended his work to be used as a practical guide to practices, he would never have written them down, violating his own cautions. Like all ancient Gurus, the written aspect of the teaching was only the tip of the iceberg, a "jolt" to the memory of the student, a reminder of the whole and not containing the whole within itself.

In Chapter One, V.11, for example, he says: "The Yogic desirous of obtaining Siddhi should keep the Hatha Yoga very secret. For it is potent when kept secret and ineffective when injudiciously revealed". In Chapter III, V.9, he says, "This should be kept secret like a casket of precious gems. It should not be spoken of to anybody as in the case of intercourse with a well born woman". This theme of secrecy runs throughout his work. He also stresses time and again, the need for the direct guidance of the Guru. Verse 78 of Chapter Three: "There is an excellent Karana by which the sun is duped. This should be learnt from the Guru and not through the study of the Shastras". In Chapter Four, V.8 he says: "Who really knows the greatness of Raja Yoga? Jnana, Mukti, Sthiti and Siddhi are obtained through the teaching of the Guru".

Thus though this text does appear to give quite detailed instructions in Asanas, Pranayama, Mudras and means of practicing Dhyana, in reality the references are very obscure and deliberately kept ambiguous, forcing the sincere aspirant not to rely on the text alone, but to seek the guidance of a qualified Master.

Hatha Yoga is the appropriate Sadhana for Kali Yuga, an age when the woman or man has lost control over his her body, emotions and sensual organs, and often lives a life hardly better than a beast. Hatha Yoga allows the practitioner to use the body as a stepping stone towards higher evolutionary levels. The body then becomes an instrument, rather than a hindrance towards achieving the noble aim of life – Moksha.

Consciousness is the key to control and intelligent Hatha Yoga makes the practitioner conscious in every cell! It may be said that the motto of Hatha Yoga is, **"Exercise to Exorcise."** Intelligent Hatha Yoga purifies body, mind and emotions of primordial reptilian / animal instincts. A rule of the human organism is *"Use it or lose it."* Hatha Yoga aids the practitioner to attain skill in right-use-ness of the body. Lower animal passions are exorcized by using the unconscious animal-like areas of the body in a conscious human manner. Essential body functions are used systematically, bringing normally autonomic functions under the conscious control of mind. In this way, the Jiva takes control of its own evolutionary trajectory. Instead of being a puppet dangling on the strings of the primordial nervous system, locked into the "4 F" Response Syndrome:-Fright, Flight, Fight or Freeze", the Jiva is able to use its cerebral cortex to consciously determine the proper response to each situation. In other words, one learns to act in the proper manner, rather than re-act in an unhealthy unconscious knee-jerk manner.

"There can be no Raja Yoga without Hatha Yoga, and no Hatha Yoga without Raja Yoga" declares Swatmarama Suri, in his *Hatha Pradipika*. When the entire array of Hatha Yoga practices such as Asana, Pranayama, Kriya, Mudras and Bandhas are practised extensively within the correct wholistic framework of Yoga as an entire life style, great peace, serenity, strength and happiness springs eternal in the heart and soul of the Yoga Sadhaka. May all attain such a state through the benevolent blessings of the great Masters who continue to guide sincere seekers on the path of Yoga.

## REFERENCES

1.  A Primer of Yoga Theory. Dr Ananda Balayogi Bhavanani. Dhivyananda Creations, Iyyanar Nagar, Pondicherry. 2008.
2.  The Forceful Yoga (being the translation of the Hathayoga Pradipika, Gheranda Samhita and Siva Samhita). Translated into English by Pancham Sinh, Rai Bahadur Srisa Chandra Vasu and Romanized and edited by Dr GP Bhatt. Mothilal Banarsidas Publishers Private Limited, Delhi. 2004.
3.  Back issues of Yoga Life, Monthly Journal of ICYER at Ananda Ashram, Pondicherry. www.icyer.com
4.  The History of Yoga from Ancient to Modern Times. Yogacharini Meenakshi Devi Bhavanani. Satya Press, Pondicherry, India. 2012.
5.  Yoga Chikitsa: Application of Yoga as a therapy. Dr Ananda Balayogi Bhavanani. Dhivyananda Creations, Iyyanar Nagar, Pondicherry. 2013

# A FEW WORDS OF ADVICE

- Always practice your hatha yoga on an empty stomach.
- Make sure there is plenty of fresh air.
- It is very important to keep yourself hydrated and hence keep sipping water.
- Try to take a gentle and progressive approach and not forceful or aggressive.
- Your space should be clean and tidy, a dusty and cluttered space is not good for your energy.
- Try to light a candle or lamp where you practice to charge the energy with some positive prana.
- Listen to your body and if it tells you to avoid something, do that or take it more carefully.
- Eat healthy and fresh food to nurture your body.
- Avoid drinking, smoking and drug mis-use, as it will be harmful if you practice hatha-yoga daily.
- Be grateful and happy for what you do and what you have.
- Hatha Yoga is not for showing off or impressing or influencing others.
- Always follow relaxation after your physical practice.

## THE SANSKRIT NAMES USED IN THIS BOOK

In modern times many of the names used for Asanas have changed. The names used in this book are authentic to the best of my knowledge and I use the terms I was taught from the authentic traditions in India my whole life. This language was said to be the language of God and it is important to use the correct terms for certain Asanas as each sound creates a vibration and an energy of its own, that is why I believe it is also important to use the Sanskrit terms when teaching Yoga authentically.

## CHAPTER 1

# SURYANAMASKAR

# 1 SURYANAMASKAR

The sun is the energy source in our solar system. As our day begins with the sunrise, so the practise of *Yogasanas* begins with the *Suryanamaskar*. *Suryanamaskar* is also known as a preparatory ladder for *Yogasanas*. *Suryanamaskar* is a vinyasa or set of various postures. The classical *Suryanamaskar* as followed by many Yoga traditions and based on ancient Indian Yoga is a set of twelve different positions, which prepare the body and mind for performing other asanas leading to raja-Yoga. In classical *Suryanamaskar*, each body posture has physical and spiritual significance - they stretch our body parts to attain flexibility, stability, strength, and endurance, as well as opening and cleansing all the naris, so our subtle energies can flow as they should for the healthy functioning of our body, mind and soul.

**SPIRITUAL POWER** A state of peace and concentration of mind is achieved by performing all the postures of *Suryanamaskar* with breath awareness or recitation of mantras. It helps in awakening the *Kundalini* if special attention is given to the *chakras*.

**BREATHING AND PRANAYAMA** In all the forward-bending positions, *rechaka* (exhalation) should be done and in all the back-bending or opening positions, *puraka* (inhalation) should be done. In certain positions, *Kumbhaka* (breath retention) and bandhas can be practised, depending on the level of sadhana.

**JOINTS, MUSCLES AND HEALTH** *Suryanamaskar* helps us to regain flexibility and mobility in our joints and muscles. It helps remove stiffness, toxins and unwanted fats from various body parts. The spine becomes supple, strong and healthy if *Suryanamaskar* is learned and practised properly.

**EFFECTS ON THE BODY SYSTEM** *Suryanamaskar* influences all the inner body systems, endocrine glands, and autonomic nervous system and helps us regain balance in our essential body functions. The *sadhaka* attains a better digestive system, circulatory system, nervous system, and so on, and hence regains overall health and well-being.

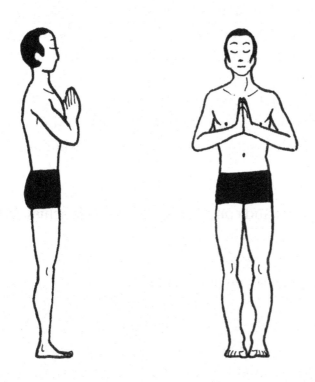

**1 SAMASTHITI** Stand straight and equally balanced on both your legs as erect as you can with ease. Join both the hands together in *Namaskar mudra* at the heart. Join your right and left energies together and connect them to your heart or spirit, reconnecting your body, mind and soul together to your heart.
Recite the mantra: *'Om Mitraya Namah'*

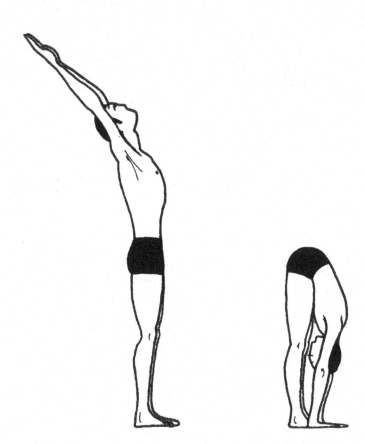

**2 TADASANA** From the first position, raise both hands upward while inhaling slowly, open your hand palms to the front, and bend backward. One should be aware of one's own strength and flexibility while performing this asana. The nerve of the legs becomes strong in this posture. This asana provides good exercise to the stomach, the back, the buttocks and the ribs.

Recite the mantra: '*Om Ravaye Namah*'

**3 HASTA PADA ASANA** Now with the out breath bend forward, keeping the spine straight, bring your hands to hold the ankle joints and gradually bring your head to your knees. You can also place the palms on the ground close to the toes. This is good exercise for the throat, neck, back, and the waist. It can also help to loosen up muscles and ligaments in the back of the thighs and legs.

Recite the mantra: '*Om Suryaya Namah*'

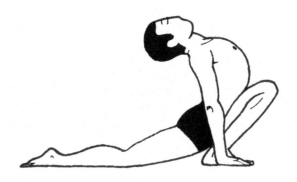

**4 ASHWA CHALANA SAPURNA** From the above position, with the in breath bend at the knees as if coming to a squatting position and step your right foot back as far as you can reach, while keeping the left foot in between both hands, which are planted on the floor. Allow the right foot to be flat with the knee resting on the ground, and arch your spine in a backbend as much as you can. This strengthens the back, hips, and knees, and opens the shoulders and heart area. The appetite increases because of the pull on the abdominal muscles. Recite the mantra: *'Om Bhanave Namah'*

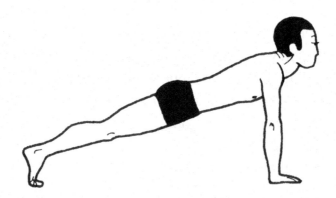

**5 SAMA TULA ASANA** With the out breath lift your right knee up, straightening your leg, and step the left foot back alongside the right. Balance on your hands and toes in a straight sloping plank position from head to feet and look forward. This is a good posture to build up strength in the shoulders, arms, hips, abdominal muscles and pelvic muscles.
Recite the mantra: *'Om Khagaye Namah'*

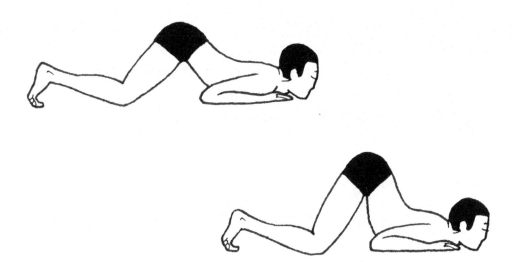

**6 SASTANGA NAMASKAR ASANA** From position *Sama Tula asana*, with the in breath bend at the elbows and place your chin, chest, knees and feet on the floor, while keeping your bottom as high as you can. This is known as *Sastanga Namaskar* as the *sadhaka* is touching eight (astanga) points on the floor. This enhances digestive capacity, re-aligns pelvic organs and muscles, opens the heart and ribcage area and loosens the neck. The mind becomes calm and leads into awakening spiritual powers.

Recite the mantra: '*Om Pushne Namah*'

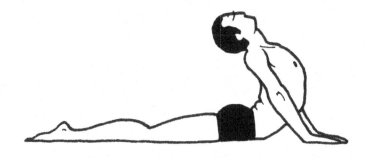

**7 BHUJANGASANA** Gradually breath out and stretch yourself into a straight position lying on your front. With the in breath, lift your head and chest up, pushing your hands into the floor, and bending back as far as you can. Keep your feet as close together as possible and keep the pelvic area on the floor. This asana strengthens the backbone and makes it flexible, widens the chest, and reduces abdominal and pelvic fat. It can control night wetting, cure constipation, and strengthen the kidneys.

Recite the mantra: '*Om Hiranayagarbhaya Namah*'

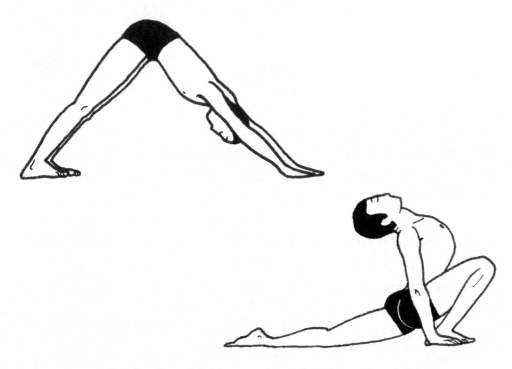

**8 MERU ASANA** Gradually with the out breath, lift up from the centre until the tailbone points up, keeping your legs and arms straight in a sloping position. Gently pushing back on your heels so that there is a straight line from hips to heels, and push the hands into the floor to make a straight line from the hips through to the shoulders to the hands, with the position being strong and grounded. This should be performed while exhaling the breath. Strengthening the feet, ankle joints, knees, hips, backbone, shoulders, arms and wrists, it works through the whole body. This also redirects our energy or *prana* from lower to higher chakras.

Recite the mantra: '*Om Marichaye Namah*'

**9 ASHWA CHALANA SAPURNA** From position 8, with the in breath come back to position 4 with the right foot coming forward in between the hands and the left leg stretched behind.
Recite the mantra: '*Om Aadityaya Namah*'

**10 PADA HASTA ASANA** With the out breath, step the left foot forward to bring both legs together and stretch them straight, bringing the head to the knees, with the hands on the floor close to the toes or feet.
Recite the mantra: '*Om Savitre Namah*'

**11 TADASANA** With the in breath, start lifting the torso, lifting your arms alongside in a big circle over your head and bend back as in position 2
Recite the mantra: '*Om Arkaya Namah*'

**12 SAMATHITI** Return back to *Namaskar mudra* in the primary position with the out breath.
Recite the mantra: '*Om Bhaskaraya Namah*'

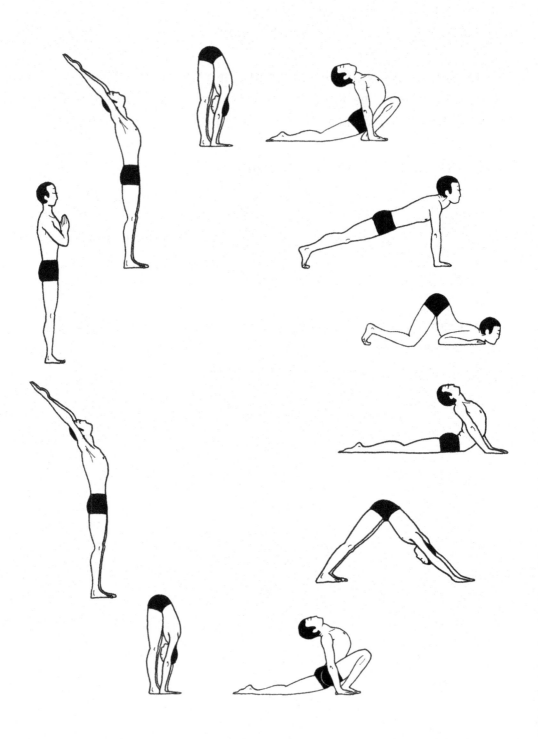

## CHAPTER 2

# STANDING POSTURES

## 2 HASTAPADA ASANA

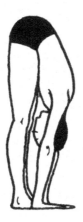

**PROCESS** Stand up straight and stretch both hands up over the head with the in breath. With the out breath bend forward slowly, keeping the legs and back straight and touch the head to the knees. Place both the palms on the floor touching the feet. Return back up with the in breath. You can repeat this as a kriya with the breath or hold the posture from 10 seconds to three minutes.

**BENEFITS**

- It stimulates muscles and ligaments connecting the lower back, hips and thighs.
- It reduces unnecessary fat around the hips and belly.
- It cures constipation and stimulates the digestive system.
- This asana enhances concentration and memory and removes mental instability and nerve weakness.

**CAUTION** Those who are suffering from ulcer, asthma, back problems or fractures should perform this asana only under strict guidance.

**SPECIAL** Very important postures for athletes and young children for loosening up and strengthening the ligaments and muscles which are tightened and stressed due to over exertion on legs, thighs, knees and hips.

This asana is also known as *Uthita Paschimottanasana*.

## 3 TADASANA

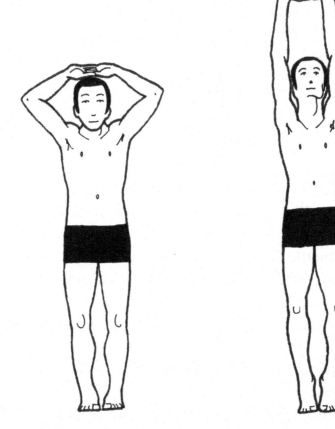

**PROCESS** Stand up straight. Interlock both hands over your head, turn your palms towards the ceiling and stretch your arms straight over your head. Lift your heels up and balance on your toes. Stretch your whole body upward as much as you can. Return back to *Samasthiti*.

**BENEFITS**
- It strengthens and lengthens the backbone.
- It refreshes the mind and rejuvenates the nervous system.
- It can help young children increase their height.
- It removes the blockages in the pores meant for perspiration, and thus cleanses skin and tissues.

**SPECIAL** This asana is called *Tadasana* because the position is like a palm tree. This is the tall position of standing. In ancient India, the great scriptures were written on palm leaves.

**DURATION:** Stay in the posture for half a minute, or repeat the asana five times with your breath.

## 4 VRIKSHASANA

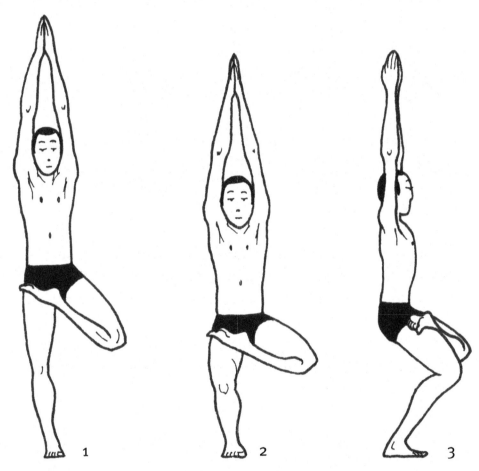

1          2          3

**PROCESS:** While standing straight, lift the left foot up and place it on top of the right thigh as in half lotus. Keeping the right leg straight, bring both hands straight over your head and join your palms together in *Anjali mudra*. Hold the posture for 30 seconds to a minute and then repeat on the other side.

### BENEFITS
- This asana develops the balance and concentration of body and mind.
- It strengthens legs and knees.
- It particularly helps children to gain control or discipline of their limbs and be more attentive.

SPECIAL *Vrikshasana* means Tree Position, representing fruits, shelter, life and growth. In ancient times, rishis or yogis used this as a meditative position as it naturally demands attentiveness and represents fruition, health and wealth in daily life.

DURATION Stay in the posture for half a minute on each side, or repeat the asana five times.

### VRIKSHASHANA VARIATIONS
1. Place one foot over the other knee or against the knee and hands, this can be in *Namaskar mudra* or *Anjali mudra*.
2. Place one foot against the other thigh and either or both variations of hand mudras. Placing Place one foot over the other thigh as in Half Lotus and either hand variation.
3. Place one foot over the other thigh, stretching hands overhead in *Anjali mudra* and slightly bending the knee as if you are trying to sit back on a chair.

## 5 HANUMANASANA

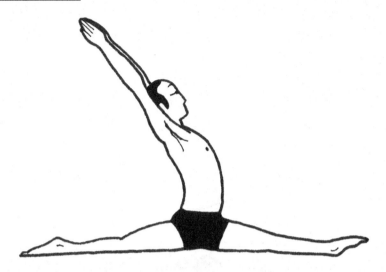

**PROCESS** Stand erect in *Samsthiti*. Bend forward to place both your hands on the floor. Bow down and put both your palms on the ground. Slowly start stretching your right leg forward and the left leg backwards, gradually coming into a full split. Keep your heels straight with your toes tucked up. Interlock both hands over your head, turn the palms upside down and stretch your hands over and gently bend backward to create an easy curve. Return back to *Pada-Hastasana* and repeat with the left leg in front and the right behind. You can hold the posture from 10 seconds to 30 seconds or more.

**BENEFITS**

- This asana gives strength and flexibility to the hips, thighs, knees, ankles, and helps loosen the muscles and ligaments around the lower back, hips, thighs and knees.
- It refines the blood and regulates blood circulation in the lower body organs.
- It aligns and shapes the hips, thighs, knees and legs.
- It refines *prana* and *naris* thus establishing health, vitality and lightness.
- It helps muscles to be flexible and removes stiffness of the back and torso.

**CAUTION** Those who have bone fractures or chronic pain or hip problems should perform this asana only under the supervision of a Yoga expert.

**SPECIAL** If practised regularly this is a very helpful posture for women to have an easy delivery. During pregnancy one should practise in a modified way or with help.

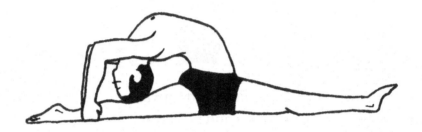

**HANUMANASANA PARIPURNA** From the above posture with the in breath bend backward to reach back to hold to your back leg with the aim of touching the leg with your head. Return back on the out breath and repeat the same on the other side.

## 6 GARUDASANA

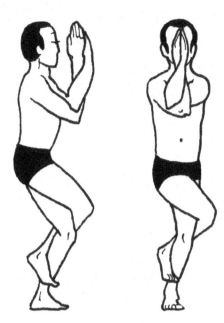

**PROCESS** Stand up straight in *Samasthiti*. Bring your right leg in front of the left and wrap it around the left leg with foot reaching behind the calf muscle of the left leg. Bring your arms in front and wrap the right arm around the left, bringing your hands in *Namaskar mudra* in front of your face. Repeat the same, changing your legs and hands.

**SPECIAL** This asana is dedicated to Garuda, the carrier of Lord Vishnu. Garuda is the symbolic character for speed, strength, devotion, and energy. In the story of '*Ramacharitramanas*'- an epic story on the life of Lord Rama', there is a mention of 'Kakabhusundi', who told this story to Garuda. A serpent Cobra and a Garuda in practical life are enemies and one preys on the other but in Hatha Yoga, Garuda and the Cobra possess equal importance. In this asana, the body gets the shape of a Garuda and connects our limbs. Twisting them around connects various naris and neurons, linking various parts of our brain together. This creates integrity, harmony and establishes co-ordination, speed, rhythm and awareness of body-mind activities.

**BENEFITS**

- This asana removes toxins and stiffness from ankles, knees, wrists and elbows and stimulates all the associated muscles.
- It brings harmony and co-ordination to the limbs by creating connections with points of the brain that regulate them.
- It increases body immunity, and concentration.

**CAUTION** Those who have fractured leg or arm bones and dislocated joints should practise this under guidance in modified asana.

**DURATION** Begin practicing this asana for a few seconds, building up to three minutes.

## 7 VATAYANASANA

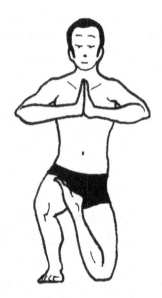

**PROCESS** Stand straight in *Samasthiti*. Place your right foot over the left thigh as in *Aradhpadmasana*. Now slowly bend your left knee to come down as if sitting on a chair, placing your right knee on the floor. Repeat the same with changed legs. From here you can practise all the *Namaskar mudra* variations.

- This asana removes toxins and stiffness from hips, thighs, knees and legs, and makes them flexible.
- It is a meditative posture and enables the sadhaka to build concentration and stability.
- It is beneficial for reproductive organs in men and women.
- It prevents and cures arthritis, pain or weakness of the waist and intestine.

**DURATION** Increase the duration of this asana from a few seconds to three minutes.

## 8 NATARAJASANA

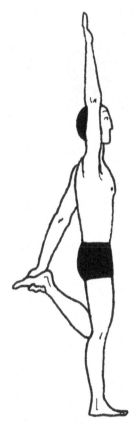

**PROCESS** Stand up erect in *Samasthiti*. Balance firmly on your right leg and then hold the left foot behind your back with the left hand.

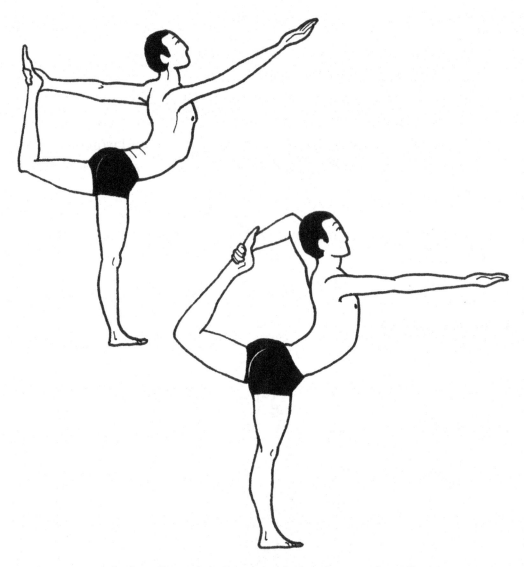

Raise your right hand straight over and slowly start bending forward, lifting and stretching your left leg behind to create a curved shape with the toes pointing over to the head. Repeat the same with the right leg behind.

**NOTE** This asana is dedicated to Lord Shiva's Dynamic form within a dancing performance. Natraj is one of the forms of Lord Shiva in dancing pose. 'Nat' means dancer, 'Raj' means king, thus the king of dancers, i.e. Lord Shiva.

## NATARAJASANA VARIATIONS

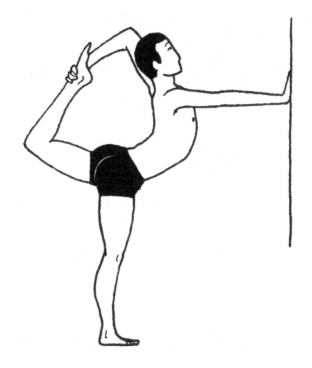

**NATARAJASANA SAPURN** Stand straight facing to a wall and place your right hand on the wall to support you, keeping an arms distance from the wall. Reach behind to hold your left leg with your left hand, stretch and pull towards your head to take the curved shape. Repeat the same with changed sides.

**NATARAJASANA PURN** As above hold your big toes behind your back and slowly pull and stretch behind to bring your toes to your head, keeping the other arm stretched in front of you facing upwards. Repeat the same one the other side.

**NATARAJASANA PARIPURN** Balancing on one leg, come to the above posture and reach back to hold to your foot with both hands on the top of your head with the elbows pointing over the head to both sides.

**BENEFITS**
- It widens the chest, strengthens arms, shoulders, knees and spine.

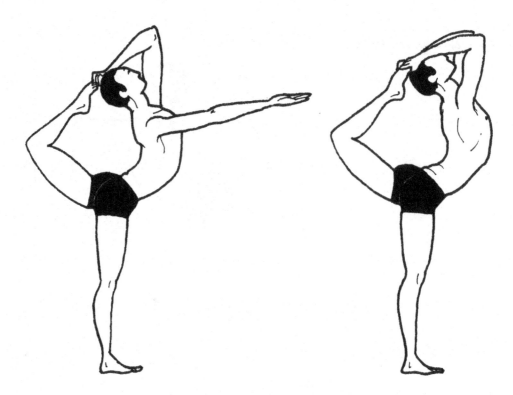

- Aligns the joints of the hands and prevents and cures rheumatism.
- It establishes physical, mental and emotional stability and vitalises the personality.
- It is beneficial for the reproductive organs and can help cure infertility in men and women. If practised in a modified way it can help pregnant women to have an easy delivery.
- The backbone becomes flexible and strong.
- It removes unnecessary fat from legs, thighs, hips and shoulders.
- It stimulates and strengthens the digestive and pelvic organs and muscles.

CAUTION Persons with weak and broken bones or joints should practise this asana carefully, under guidance.

DURATION Perform this asana from a few seconds to three minutes.

## 9 MURGASANA

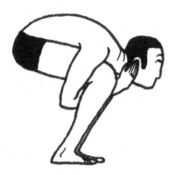

**PROCESS** Stand up straight keeping hip distance between both the feet. Gradually, bend forward from the knees, bringing your head towards them. Bring your hands under your thighs from behind to hold onto your ears and look in front, while gazing on your eyebrows.

**NOTE** This asana is very important for increasing attentiveness, concentration and memory of students. Therefore, in schools the teachers used to use this posture whenever they found students laking in attentiveness and concentration.

**BENEFITS**
- This asana increases attentiveness, concentration and memory.
- It removes unnecessary fat, flatulence, indigestion and constipation.
- It stimulates and strengthens the reproductive organs.
- It strengthens kidneys and balances adrenal glands.
- It helps the nervous system to function properly.

**CAUTION** Those who suffer with dizziness should perform this asana under guidance.

**DURATION** Begin it for a few seconds and build up to three minutes.

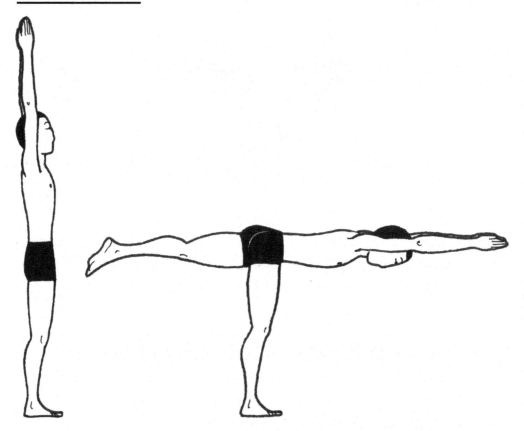

**PROCESS** Stand straight in *Samasthiti*. Lift both your hands over the head, palms facing each other. Now slowly bend forward from the torso, lifting your left leg back and come to a position where both hands, head, back, hips and left leg are in same straight line. Repeat the same while balancing on the right leg.

**NOTE** *Eka Pada Asana* resembles a *Tula* (a weighing scale) where both the weighing pans remain balanced on a single support. Some Yoga experts also call it *Tulasana*.

**BENEFITS**
- This asana helps achieve strength, flexibility and endurance of legs, knees, hips, shoulders and back.

- It removes abdomen disorders, fat and toxins.
- This asana helps achieving physical, mental and emotional balance.
- This asana strengthen core and pelvic muscles.

**CAUTION** This asana should be performed in combination with *Pad Prasar and Hanumanasana*.

**DURATION** Perform this asana from a few seconds to three minutes.

## 11 UTTHIT VIPREETPASCHIMOTTANASANA

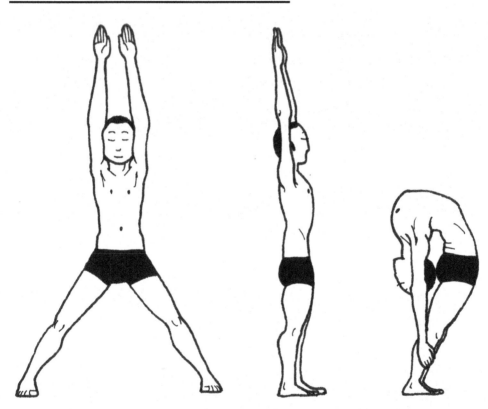

**PROCESS** Stand up straight while keeping both legs hip width apart. Slowly lift both your hands upwards with the in breath. Breathe out and then with the next in breath bend back to reach back and hold your shinbones, with the head touching the buttocks. Return back up with the in breath.

**BENEFITS**
- This asana is beneficial for the stomach, liver, kidneys and adrenal glands.
- This is another extreme back bend and strengthens back, hips, shoulder, thighs and knees.
- It refines bool, prana and naris and brings harmony to the pancha-kosha and prevents all sorts of psycho-somatic diseases.
- It prepares the spinal cord and sushumna for the entry of the *Kundalini* energy.

**CAUTION** It is an extreme back bend and one must master *Chakrasana*, *Bhujangasana* and *Shalbhasana* before practising this posture. This asana should be practised under the supervision of a Yoga expert.

**DURATION** Practise from a few seconds to half a minute or more.

## 12 UTTHIT TRIVIKRAMASANA

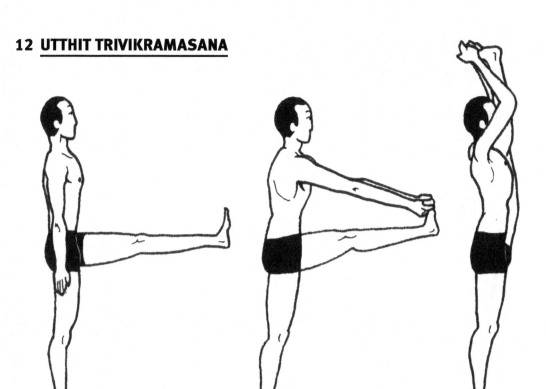

**PROCESS** Stand up straight and lift up the left leg in front. Now hold your toes with both hands and stretch your leg over your head. Maintain the balance on your straight right leg. Repeat the same on switched legs.

**BENEFITS**

- This asana stretches and stimulates hips, pelvic organs and muscles, lower back and ligaments through the legs.
- It prepares for healthy pregnancy and helps in easy delivery if practised before conception.
- This asana is beneficial for strengthening the abdominal, pelvic and core areas.
- It stimulates the nervous system and increases concentration, balance of mind and memory.
- This asana improves blood circulation in the feet, legs, thighs, and waist.

**CAUTION** Persons with back problems and weak joints should perform this asana under guidance.

**DURATION** Begin it for a few seconds and try to master for three minutes.

## 13 HASTHA ASANA

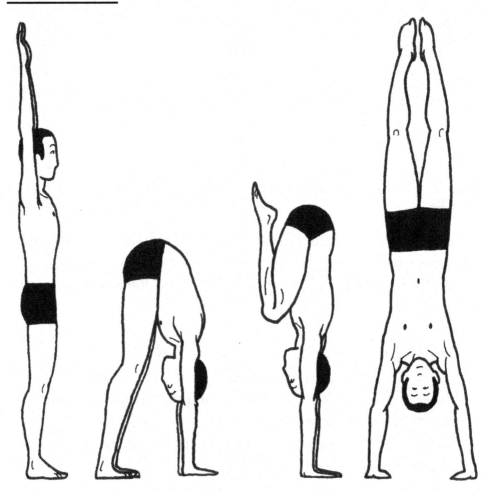

**PROCESS** Stand up straight in *Samasthiti*. Lift your hand over your head with the in breath. With the out breath slowly bend forward and place both the palms firmly on the floor, hip width apart.

Slightly bend from the knees and then lift your whole body straight over your head with straight arms.

- This asana prevents and cures digestive problems, waist and back problems, leprosy, jaundice, enlarged testicles, and sexual disorders.
- It stimulates the nervous system, balances the autonomic nervous system and increases memory power.
- It makes the backbone flexible and strong.
- This asana strengthens shoulders and the chest.

CAUTION This asana should be practised only after expertise *Vrashchikasana*. Persons with weak joints or bones, high blood pressure, heart problems and tuberculosis of bones should perform this asana under guidance.

DURATION Begin it for a few seconds and try to build up for three minutes.

## 14 RATHACHARIYA ASANA

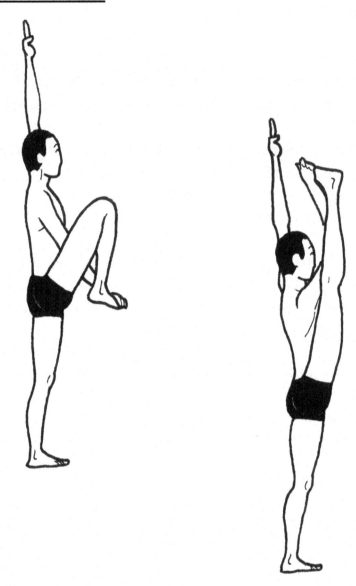

**PROCESS** Stand straight in *Samasthiti*. Balance firmly on your left leg and slowly lift your right leg up with a bent knee. Now hold your foot or toes with the right hand and stretch your left hand straight up over your head. With a deep in breath stretch your right leg straight in front and hold your posture. Return back and follow the same with changed legs and hands.

## RATHACHARIYA VARIATIONS

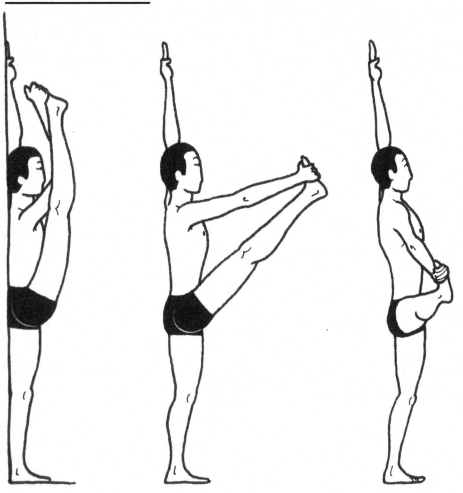

**RATHACHARIYA SALAMBA** In the beginning you might like to stand with your back resting against a wall. Bring your right leg in front and hold your foot with the right hand with the left hand over your head resting against the wall to support. Now stretch your right leg in front and hold to your posture. Repeat the same with changed sides.

**RATHACHARIYA PURNA** As in rathachariya, stretch your leg in front and bring your foot over and in front of the head, keeping the leg straight and with the left hand over the head in *Pataka mudra*. Repeat the same with changed sides.

**RATHACHARIYA PRAVRITTI ASANA** As in *Rathachariya asana,* holding your right foot with the right hand, with the left hand pointing up over your head stretch and open your right leg out to the right side to waist height and hold your posture. Repeat the same with changed sides.

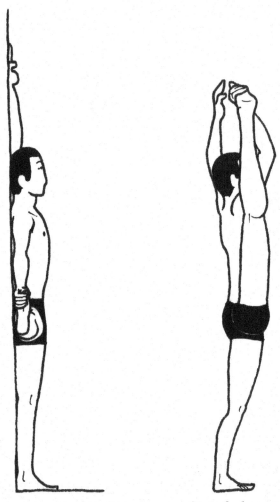

**RATHACHARIYA PRAVRITTI SALAMBA** Stand close to the wall with the left hand firmly placed on the wall over your head. Hold your right foot with the right hand and stretch and open your leg out to the right side and hold your posture. Repeat the same on the other side.

**RATHACHARIYA PRAVRITTI SAPURNA** Come to *Rathachariya Pravritti asana* and stretch your right leg further up to bring your foot and hand in line with the left hand to your side, with the left hand pointing to your foot in *Pataka mudra*. Repeat the same with the other side.

**BENEFITS**
- It helps builds balance, flexibility and stability in standing positions.
- It opens hips, stretches and stimulates muscles and ligaments connected to legs, thighs, hips, pelvis, abdomen and back.
- This series stimulates and strengthens abdominal and pelvic organs and improves health and vitality.
- It eradicates lethargy, heaviness, lack of interest or energy and weaknesses of body and mind.
- It increases attentiveness, concentration and memory.

**DURATION** starting from a few seconds, the whole series should be practised for five minutes or more for the desired benefits.

**CAUTION** If you are suffering with chronic back or hip problems, practise under guidance of a Yoga expert.

## 15 PADOTTANASANA

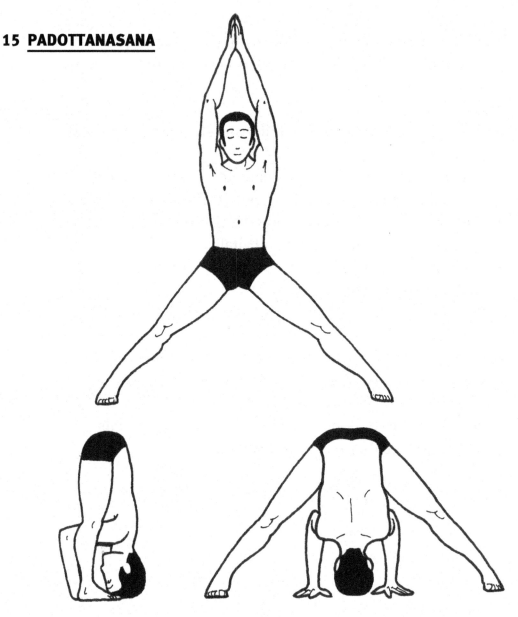

**PROCESS** Stand straight in the *Sama-Shiti-asana*, slowly move the legs apart as much as you can. Raise both the hands straight over the head. Align both the hands with the head and spine and without arching the back slowly bend in front and place both the palms in the middle of both the feet in the same line. Lower your head and try to place the head in middle of the palms while keeping your spine straight. This is *Padottana-asana*.

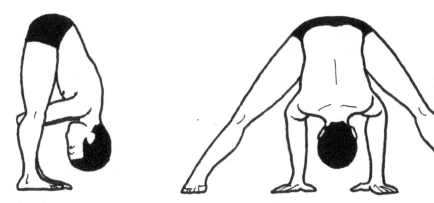

**PADOTTANASANA SAPURN** From a wide open leg position come forward to place your hands on the floor in the middle and in line with both feet and let your head come down, hanging towards the floor.

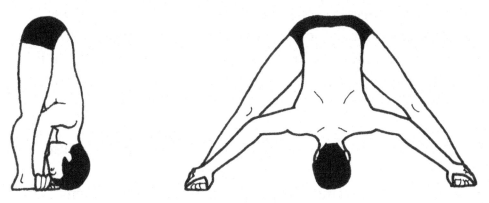

**PADOTTANASANA PURNA** From *Padottanasana* once you feel comfortable, stretch your arms to the sides and hold your ankle joints.

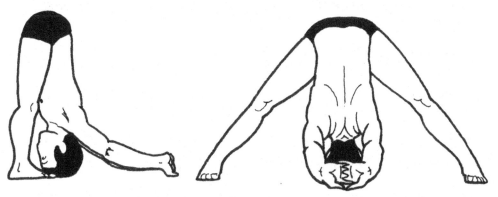

**PADOTTANASANA PARIPURNA** From *Padottanasana*, bring your arms over your back, interlock both hands, turn your palms inside out and stretch out. If it's too uncomfortable you can also join your hands in *Namaskar mudra* straight out over the back.

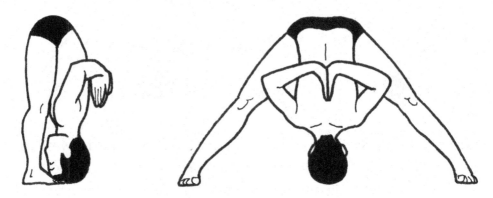

**PADOTTANASANA SAMPURNA** Come to *Padottanasana* with your head resting on the floor and join your hands in *Hamsa mudra* (reverse *Namaskar mudra* behind the back). Hold your posture while holding *Mahabandha*.

**BENEFITS**
- This series strengthens back, hip joints, pelvic muscles and abdominal muscles.
- It redirects blood and energy upwards to the heart and head, thus prevents and cures problems associated with the heart and head.
- It stretches and stimulates all the abdominal and pelvic organs and thus prevents and cures abdominal, digestive and pelvic health issues.
- It builds core and pelvic strength.

**DURATION** This series should be practised for five minutes or more.

**CAUTION** Practise under strict guidance if you suffering with hip, or back injuries, heart diseases or blood pressure.

**SPECIAL** This asana should be followed with a back bend like *Chakrasana* or *Dhanurasana* and a side stretch like *Ardha Chandrasana*.

## 16 UTHITA TRIKONASANA

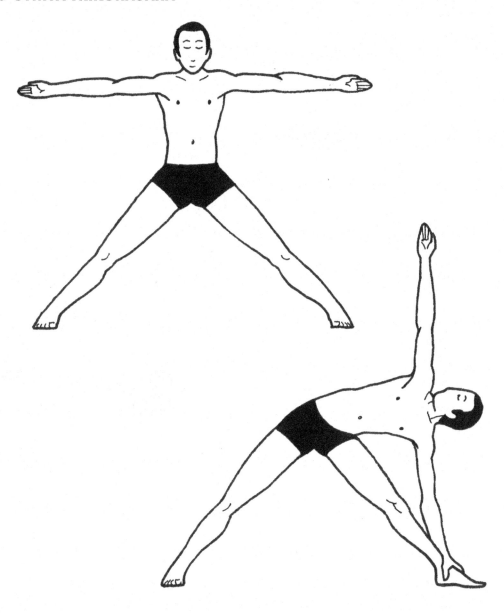

**TRIKONASANA** Stand straight with the legs wide opened. Now stretch both your arms straight up to your shoulders. Come over to the right side and place the back of your right hand against the right leg and foot, while the left hand points over to the ceiling. Repeat the same with left side.

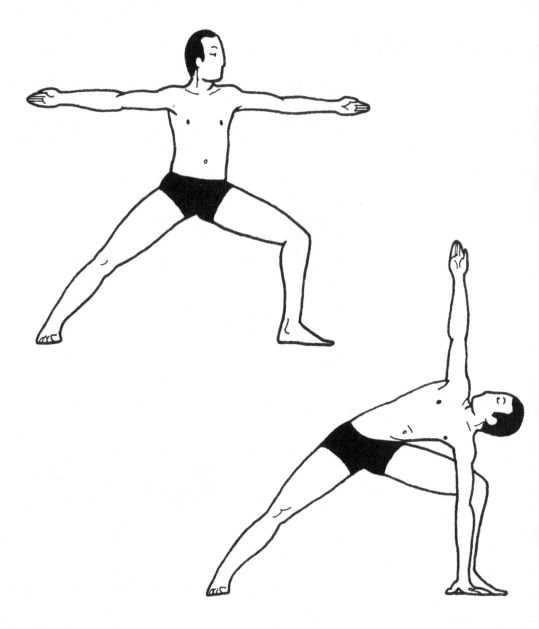

**TRIKONASANA PRAVRITTI** Stand straight with the legs wide open and with arms stretched straight up to the shoulders. Turn your right foot out to the side and bend your right leg to 90 degrees in *Veerasana*. Place your right hand on the floor in front of the foot with the left hand pointing over to the ceiling. You can also place the right hand on the floor over your leg, outside of your foot. Repeat the same with switched sides.

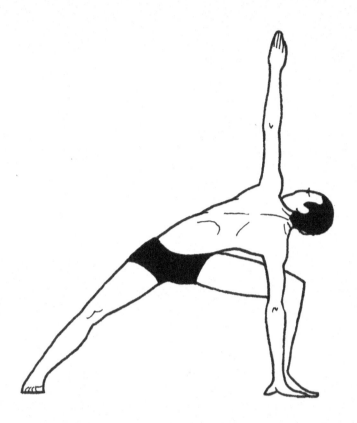

**TRIKONASANA PROVRITTI** Come to *Veerasana* as above. Now bring both your hands parallel to your shoulders as in the *Veerasana* variation. Now come down and place your left hand on the floor close to the right foot with the right hand pointing over to the ceiling. Repeat the same to other side.

## CHAPTER 3

# ASANA PRACTICES AND SEQUENCES FROM VAJRASANA

## 17 SUPTA VAJRASANA

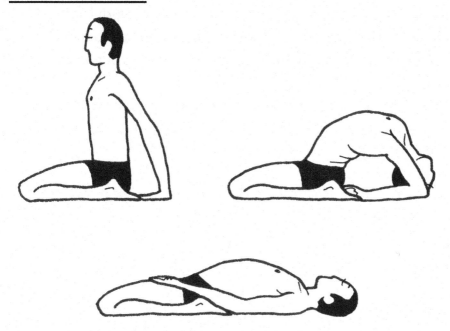

**PROCESS** Choose one of the variations of *Vajrasana*. Gently bend back, placing your hands on the floor behind your feet. Bend further back to place your elbows down and supporting with arms and elbows gradually place your head down on the floor. If possible you can bring closer to the floor, pushing the head further over. Finally place your hands on the thighs while keeping elbows on the floor. Supta means lying down and this position is known as *Supta Vajrasana*.

### BENEFITS
- It stimulates and strengthens the digestive system.
- Pushing back on the hips against heels stimulates the kidneys and adrenal glands to improve health and well being.
- This asana is a complete stretch for the backbone and maintains spinal health. It also stimulates all the nerves originating from the spinal column reaching out and in. This reactivates them as well as the bio-memory of the body's cells.
- It increases concentration and memory.

- The body, face and skin become radiant.
- It stretches the backbone. Therefore, dislocated vertebral columns resume their normal position and the backbone becomes healthy and strong if practised under supervision.

**CAUTION** Patients suffering from tuberculosis or chronic backbone problems should perform this asana only under strict supervision in modified ways to start.

**DURATION** Start for a few seconds, eventually this asana should be performed for three to five minutes for better results as a complete series.

## 18 LAGHU VAJRASANA

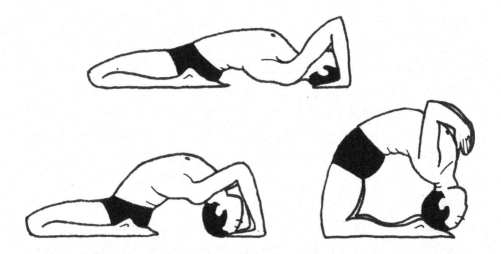

**PROCESS** From *Supta Vajrasana* bring your hands over your head on the floor and place both palms down on the floor with palms and fingers pointing inward to the shoulders. Now slowly lift your shoulders and chest up to bring the top of the head to the floor. Push further up from the centre of your spine, lifting your bottom up also and gradually placing your head on your feet. You can keep your hands over for support or if possible bring the hands over the heart into *Namaskar mudra*. Slowly return back to a relaxed position. One can hold this posture from a few seconds to one minute.

**BENEFITS** Along with all the above with *Supta Vajrasana*, this version stimulates and strengthens the backbone, neck, arms, shoulders, thighs and knees and removes toxins accumulated in these areas. It establishes health, vitality and attentiveness in children and prevents all sorts of psycho-somatic disorders.

**CAUTION** Those suffering from tuberculosis, chronic backbone problems, ulcer, neck or shoulder injuries should perform this asana only under strict supervision.

## 19 SHASHANKASANA

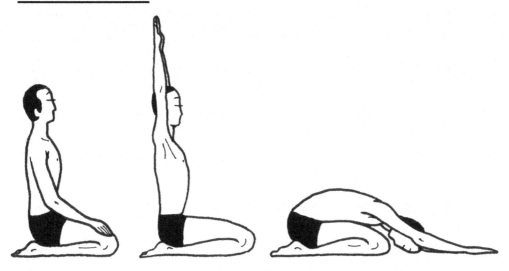

**PROCESS** Sit up in *Vajrasana*. Lift both hands over head with the in breath and as you exhale, place both palms on the floor with the arms stretched on the ground over your head and the forehead resting on the floor. You can repeat this as a kriya with breath, or hold the posture for between 30 seconds and a few minutes.

**BENEFITS**

- This is especially beneficial for relaxing the heart and nervous system.
- It strengthens the muscles of the hands and feet as well as the ribs and waist if repeated as a kriya.
- It is beneficial for the digestive system, liver, and appetite.
- It enhances appetite capacity.

**SPECIAL** This asana massages the heart and helps reduce unnecessary fat. It normalises blood circulation. It removes poisonous elements accumulated in the joints of the hands and the feet.

**CAUTION** Persons with displaced vertebra or back problems should practise this asana only under the supervision of a Yoga expert.

**NOTE** Rabbits are well known for their attentiveness and speed. A rabbit can be attentive even while it is sleeping and with minimal stimulus will charge up and run to escape danger. *Shashankasana* can help children to relax and be attentive.

## 20 USTRASANA

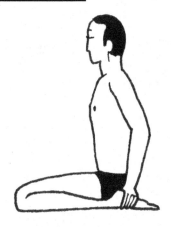 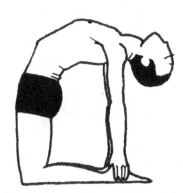

**PROCESS** Come to a kneeling position while keeping your feet flat and hip width apart. Place your buttocks on the floor in the middle of your feet and place your hands on your heels. Now slowly lift up your buttocks while pointing your navel and chest upwards and head hanging behind. You can also bend back from the kneeling position and reach down to hold your heels while creating an arch with the thighs, spine and chest. Hold your posture for few deep breaths.

### USTRASANA VARIATIONS

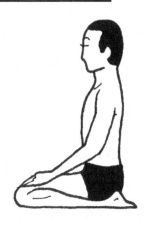 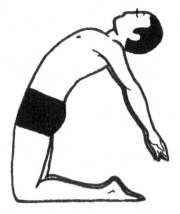

**USTRASANA SAPURNA** Sit straight in *Vajrasana*. With the in breath come up to kneeling and bend back while opening your arms back and return back with the out breath to sitting position.

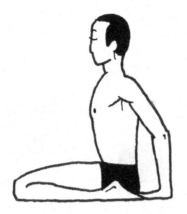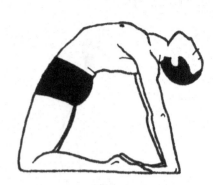

**USTRASANA PURNA** Sit in *Vajrasana* and place both your hands on the floor behind your feet with your fingers touching your toes. Now while keeping your hands on the floor, lift up your buttocks and stretch your backbone into a back bend. You can hold the posture for a few breaths or repeat a few rounds with breath.

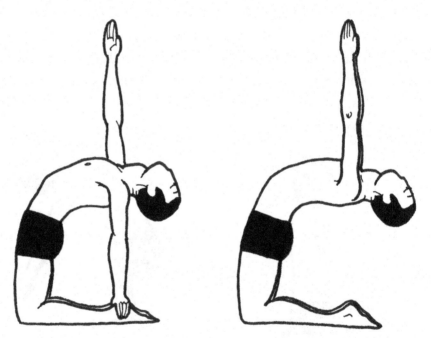

**USTRASANA PURNA** Come to *Ustrasana* and then slowly lift your right hand and bring it over your chest pointing straight up. Slowly bring your left hand up too and join them together in *Agra mudra* over your heart.

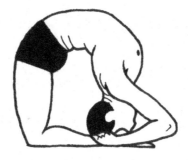

**USTRASANA PARIPURNA** Come to *Ustrasana* and then slowly bend back to place your head on your heels and let your elbows point over your head.

**BENEFITS**

- This asana strengthens the back bone, stimulates the nervous system and increases concentration and memory.
- It removes unnecessary fat and bloated stomach and resumes a normal shape.
- It prevents and cures arthritis, back pain, and slip discs.
- It widens the chest and strengthens lungs and heart.
- It strengthens the neck and balances the thyroid.

**CAUTION** Those who suffer from epilepsy, dizziness and high blood pressure should practise this asana in the presence of a Yoga expert.

**DURATION** This asana series should be performed for at least five minutes for the best results.

## 21 KUNDALINI ASANA

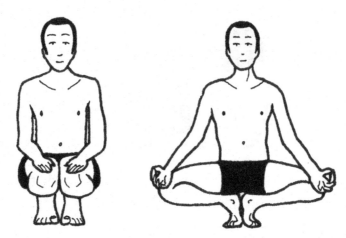

**PROCESS** Sit straight on a mat. Tuck your toes on the floor and sit up on your heels. Slowly open your knees out wide, keeping heels together. Place both hands on knees in *Jnana mudra*.

### BENEFITS

- This asana strengthens ankles and knees and opens hips and pelvic muscles to achieve flexibility.
- This asana is beneficial for men and women in improving sexual health.
- It refines and regulates lower energy to higher energy. Therefore it is one of the important postures in cleansing and transforming the personality.
- This asana puts stimulating pressure on the toes and so stimulates the brain and nervous system.

**CAUTION** Those who have ankle or knee problems should perform this asana under guidance.

**DURATION** Begin practicing from a few seconds and master for up to three minutes.

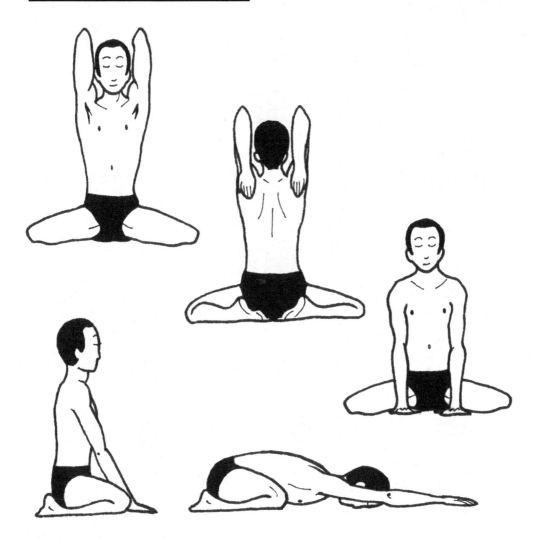

**MANDUAKA ASANA SAPURN** Come to a kneeling position. Make your feet flap so that both the toes keep touching each other and heels apart as much as possible. Sit down, placing your buttocks in between the two soles on the ground. Now stretch your knees away from each other, as far as possible. Raise your hands over the head and fold, place both the palms firmly behind the shoulders and elbows pointing over the head. Now place your hands on the floor and walk or slide them forward to come flat down on the floor in front of your chest and head.

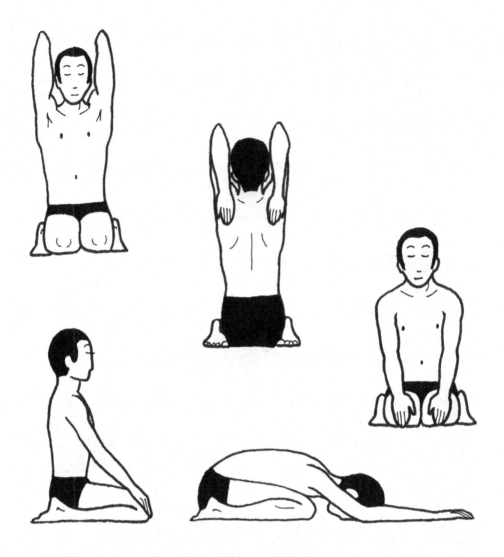

**MANDUKA ASANA PURNA** From a kneeling position, open your feet wide enough so you can place your bottom on the floor in the middle of your feet with your soles facing upward. Repeat the rest same as above.

**BENEFITS**

*Manduka* is the sanskrita term, which means frog. Thus it can be translated as frog posture or frog mudra. This is categorized in both asana and mudra. This is one of the most important practises in yoga. It seals the energy circuits in both the soles and the palms, which is why it is also known as a mudra.

- This mudra transforms the lower energy to the higher spiritual energy. This also aligns the upper chest and shoulders and stretches the upper lungs. So, it is also good for upper chest breathing problems. It helps in the opening of the swadhisthana chakra in the process of *Kundalini* awakening.
- This mudra is extremely good for the heart, lungs, shoulders and the chest area. It stimulates the blood circulation in the pelvic region and thus very good for pregnancy and for women who wish to conceive. This is extremely helpful in practicing chastity and develops tremendous energy and vitality in whole body. All kinds of male and female sexual disorders are prevented and cured by the regular practise of this mudra.
- It provides good massage to the whole pelvic region and thus stimulates and balances the functions of the kidneys, adrenal glands, gonads, uterus, and pelvic muscles. This stimulates proper flow of the blood in this region. It also helps in purifying the blood properly by activating the kidneys. It prevents the chances of developing cancer in the uterus, gonads, and large intestine.

## 23 VAJRA VEERA ASANA

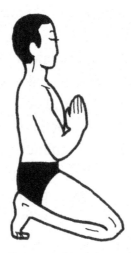

The word vajra means diamond or thunderbolt and the word veera means the warrior or the brave one. This group of asanas is designed to make your body, mind and emotions steady, firm and strong to fight and over come the day to day hassles of life. This also helps one to overcome obstacles on the yogic path.

Our soles are also full of the reflex centers of all the essential organs in the body. Acupuncture and acupressure treat most of the diseases by stimulating and balancing these reflexogenic centers in the sole.

Our big toes and heels are joined with the cranial nerves and sitting in any of *Veeriya asanas* stimulates them. Thus this group of asanas removes all the mental problems related to thoughts, emotions, concentration, and memory. They stimulate all the essential organs and endocrine glands, thus keeping you physically, mentally and emotionally healthy and balanced.

Various hand mudras rejuvenate your aura and pranic energy or the pranic sheath protecting your body. They also keep all the five koshas in proper alignment, leading to a balanced, peaceful and healthy life.

**SPECIAL** In this asana, you can use many of the hands mudras like *Anjali mudra, Kailash mudra, Agra-mudra, Namaskar mudra,* etc.

**VAJRA VEERA ASANA** Like *Vajrasana*, sit on your heels, keeping them close and both the feet straight and only the toes placed firmly on the ground. Keep the knees on the ground to keep the body in balance. Most of the body weight should be on the toes of both the legs and the knees should be passive. Try to keep the spine straight and hands in *Anjali mudra* or any of the *Namaskar mudra*.
As the name tends, warrior, braveness and courage is developed by practicing this asana. This is extremely good for stimulating the cranial nerves and opening the channels of prana flow in the brain.

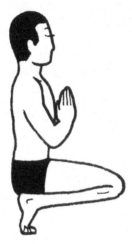

**VAJRA VEERA ASANA PURN** Like *Vajrasana* sit on your heels while keeping them close and both the feet straight with the toes placed firmly on the ground. Your body weight should be spread across all the toes. Your knees should be high from the ground in a straight line with your thighs. Try to keep the spine straight and hands in *Anjali mudra* or any of the *Namaskar mudra*.

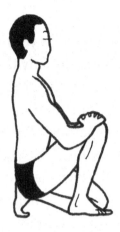

**VAJRA VEERIYA ASANA** Like the *Vajra Veera asana* now try to balance your body weight on one straight foot with placing the respective buttock on it. Place the second foot close to the knee of the first leg on the ground in the inner side. Keep this knee as high as possible. Clasp both the hands on your up side knee. Try to keep the spine straight. Practise thesame with the changed legs.

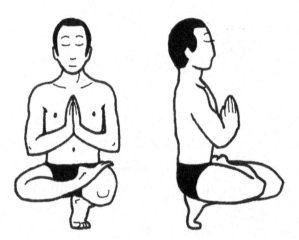

**BRAHMACHARYA ASANA** Like the *Vajra Veera asana*, now try to balance your body weight on one straight foot, while placing the respective buttock on it. Place the second foot on the thigh of the other leg close to the root of the leg. Keep the knee of the lower leg high in a straight line with its thigh. In the beginning it may be not easy, but regular practise develops tremendous concentration, power, awareness and steadiness. Try to keep the spine straight. Practise the same with changed legs. You may keep your hands in any of the *Namaskar mudras*.

## CHAPTER 4

# ASANA PRACTICES AND SEQUENCES FROM UTTANASANA (LEGS OUTSTRETCHED)

## 25 JANUSIRASANA

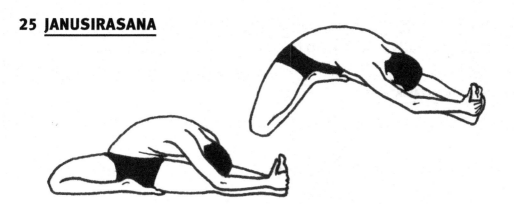

**PROCESS** Sit down on your mat stretching both legs forward. Bend the right leg and place your foot against the left inner thigh close to the groin. Now reach forward to hold the left foot with both hands, keeping the spine straight and gradually place your head over your knee as far as you can reach with the out breath. You can hold this posture for a few deep breaths or repeat it three to five times with your breath, stretching forward with the out breath and returning back to sitting up with the in breath. Repeat the same on the other side.

### BENEFITS

- This asana cures abdominal and pelvic organs, particularly the liver, kidney, and reproductive organs.
- This is beneficial for both men and women in redirecting sexual energy into spiritual energy.
- This is beneficial in preventing hay-fever and digestive problems, and in awakening the *Kundalini*. It equally affects the digestive system.
- This asana helps to bring legs, thighs and hips into good shape and alignment.
- It removes stiffness and toxins from the whole body.

**CAUTION** Students suffering from ulcers or chronic problems of the spine, asthma or tuberculosis should perform this asana only under supervision of an expert Yoga teacher.

**DURATION** In the beginning one should practise this posture for a few seconds, gradually working up to holding it for up to five minutes.

**JANUSIRASASANA VARIATIONS**

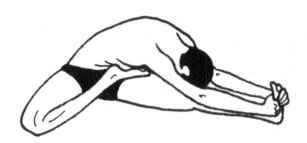

**JANUSIRASANA PURNA** Place your right foot on top of the left thigh and repeating the same as above. Repeat the same on the other side.

**JANUSIRASANA PARIPURNA** Place your right foot on top of the left thigh and hold the above posture, while holding the breath out and simultaneously holding the three *bandhas* together as long as you can hold your breath out. Release with the out breath and repeat the same on the other side.

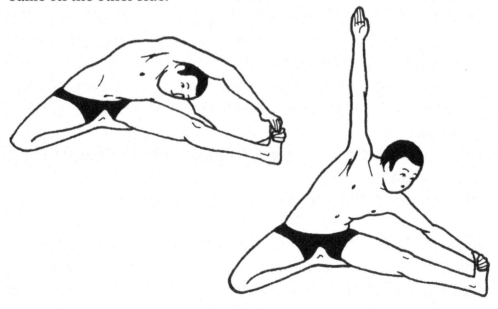

**JANUSIRASANA PARIVRATTA** Place the right foot against the left thigh or on top of the left thigh, then stretch the left hand over your left leg and hold your foot or toes. Lift your right hand over your head, twisting to the right side. Gradually, with the in breath, let the left side of the torso come down and rest on the left leg, enabling you to reach the left foot with your right hand too, looking out to the right through your arms. Repeat the same on the other side. One can hold the posture from 10 seconds to thre

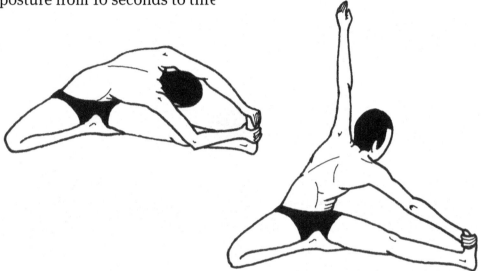

**JANUSIRASANA PRAVRITTI** As above, this time with the in breath reach down to hold to your left foot with the right hand, and twist as deep as you can to place your right side down onto the left leg and reach down to hold the left foot with the left hand too over your head. Reverse the twist to variation 3. Come to a relaxed position with the out breath. Repeat the same on the other side. These variations in addition to the above benefits are also good for the waist, spine and nervous system. They helps cleanse the *naris* and *pancha kosha* and awaken the *Kundalini*.

**DURATION:** In the beginning one can hold these postures for a few seconds, and gradually the complete series one by one can be practised for five minutes.

## 26 <u>PASCHIMOTTANASANA</u>

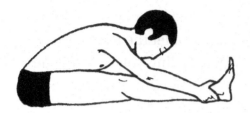

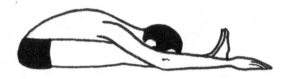

**PROCESS:** Sit straight with both legs stretched straight in front. Lift both arms straight over your head with the in breath. With the out breath, stretch forward moving from the lower back, keeping the spine straight, and reach down to hold both feet. Keep your spine straight and your chin up and take a deep breath. Now with the out breath bring your chest and head down to your legs and let your hands rest on the ground to either side. Come back to sitting with the arms stretched over the head with the in breath, and relax your arms with the out breath. You can repeat this as a kriya in the beginning for lengthening your spine and attaining flexibility, and gradually aim to hold for three minutes.

**BENEFITS:**
- This asana strengthens the spine and rejuvenates it. Your spine attains strength, flexibility and suppleness.
- This asana is beneficial in disorders like diabetes, flabby belly, flatulence, backache, and constipation and helps to preserve celibacy.

- Beneficial in diseases like leucorrhoea and menstrual disorders in women and sexual disorders in men.
- It stimulates and recharges the nervous system, and increases memory and concentration.
- It strengthens the kidneys and the digestive system.
- It removes mental instability and nerve weakness.
- This asana increases vitality and cures infertility.

CAUTION Those who are suffering from ulcers, asthma, or tuberculosis should perform this asana only under guidance. This asana should be performed only on an empty stomach.

SPECIAL The word *paschim* means the back. In this asana, the complete back is stretched. Therefore, it is called *Paschimottanasana*. It is also called *Ugrasana* or *Brahamcharayasana*.
In animals, the backbone is horizontal and the heart, being beneath the backbone, keeps them healthy and gives them extraordinary powers of endurance.
In human beings, the backbone is vertical and the heart is not beneath it, so we can feel tired quickly and fall prey to heart disease. In *Paschimottanasana*, the backbone is kept horizontal and the heart comes beneath it. This provides necessary massage to the heart, backbone, and the stomach.

DURATION: In the beginning do it for a few seconds, eventually the whole chain of this asana should be performed in five minutes or more.

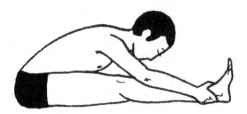

**PASCHIMOTTANASANA SAPURNA** In the beginning as above one might simply try to hold the legs close to the ankle joints or hold the feet and bend forward as much as possible, keeping the legs straight. If this is too painful you can ease your knees and stretch again and repeat.

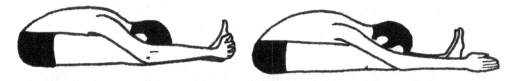

**PASCHIMOTTANASANA PURNA** Once you can touch your head to your knees as above in the main postures, then you can try to interlock your fingers and stretch your hands over your feet and hold the posture.

**PASCHIMOTTANASANA PARIPURNA** From *Paschimottanasana Purna* you can stretch your arms further and join hands in *Namaskar mudra* over your feet on the floor, maintaining the rest of the posture.

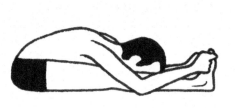 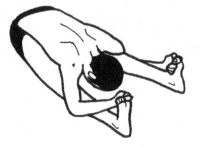

**PASCHIMOTTANASANA PADANGUSTHA** Sit straight with your legs stretched forward, hip width or about one foot apart. Now stretch forward to hold the big toes with index fingers and thumbs. Pull forward to bring your chest and head down on the floor with your elbows resting on the floor to either side of the legs.

**PASCHIMOTTANASANA MUDRA** As above in *Padangustha,* you hold it while holding the breath out and *Mahabandha.* This posture is of special significance in *Kundalini* awakening and *Nari Suddhi.*

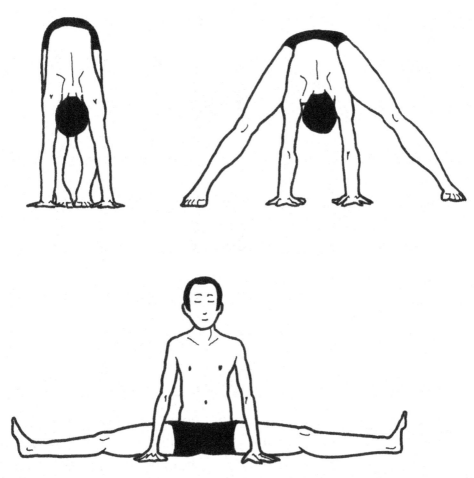

**PASCHIMOTTANASANA PADAPRASAR** Stand straight in *Samasthiti*. Place your hands down on the floor and then stretch both your legs out to either side, coming to a full side split.

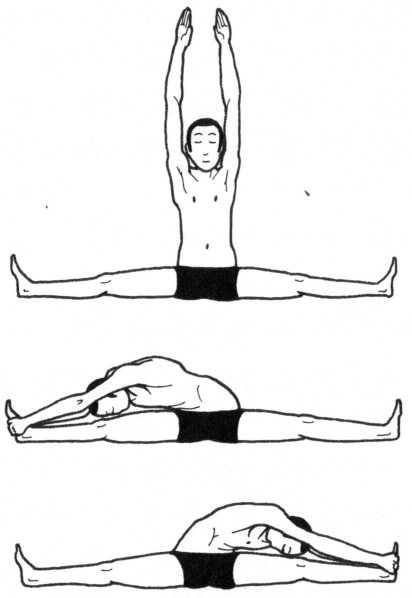

Now stretch both your arms over your head and gradually stretch over your left leg with the out breath, placing your chest over the thigh and head over the knee. You can hold the posture as long as you can hold your breath out. Return back to the centre with arms stretched over the head with the in breath and repeat the same over the left side.

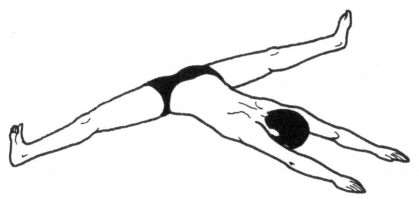

Finally stretch in front aiming to come forward and place your chest, shoulders and chin flat on floor, keeping your arms stretched overhead. This posture should be done as a complete series of stretches.

This is one of the advance postures to cleanse our naris, stimulate the nervous system, open the hips, stretch the spine, and lengthen muscles and ligaments throughout the body from toes to head. Its also has a very high importance in spiritual awakening. With young children as they are naturally flexible this can help them to attain a tremendous amount of self confidence and control over their body, mind and limbs, and develop concentration and attentiveness. One needs to be very skilful to be trained in this posture and it needs patience and care to avoid injuries or harm.

## 27  KURMASANA

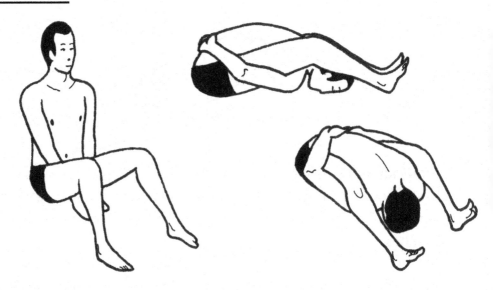

**PROCESS** Sit down with your legs stretched forwards, opened hip width. Bend your knees slightly to place your hands under your legs reaching behind your bottom to interlock them. Now with the out breath, stretch forward to place your chest and chin down on the floor. You can hold your posture with the bandhas or repeat it five times with the breath.

### BENEFITS

- This asana is beneficial for backache, headache, and neck ache.
- It stimulates and strengthens the kidneys.
- It prevents diabetes, and removes excess fat from the belly and hip area.
- It is beneficial for nervous disorders and concentration problems.
- It helps preserve and redirect sexual energy to higher energies for health and vitality.
- It plays an active role in awakening the *Kundalini*.
- It removes toxins accumulated around the knees, thighs, hips and spine and brings flexibility. It removes stiffness from the whole body.

**CAUTION** Those who are suffering from ulcer, asthma, tuberculosis or bone fractures or dislocated joints should perform this asana only under strict guidance. This asana should be performed only on an empty stomach. Persons suffering from chronic backache should perform this asana very cautiously.

**SPECIAL** This asana calms the mind. The body assumes the posture of a tortoise, hence it is called *Kurmasana*. Just like the turtle hides all its limbs in case of danger, a yogi learns to master the senses and closes them to flow inward whenever needed.

**DURATION** In the beginning do this posture for a few seconds. Eventually for the full benefit this series of asana should be performed for five minutes.

**KURMASANA VARIATIONS**

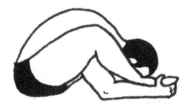

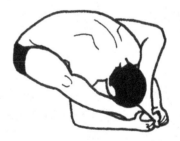

**KURMASANA SAPURNA** In a sitting position bring both your feet together and push your feet a few steps forward, tuck your hands under your forelegs and hold your feet together. Now with the out breath come forward and place your head or chin on your feet. You can hold this from 10 seconds to three minutes or repeat five rounds with the breath.

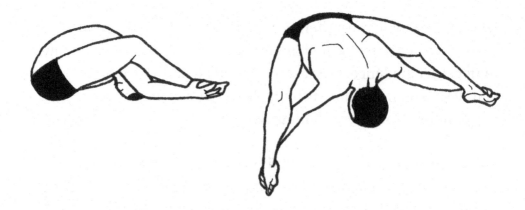

**KURMASANA PURNA** From the above position open your legs out and in front as far as you can whilst keeping your hands tucked under your legs and holding the feet. Now with the out breath come forward and try to place your chest and chin on the floor. You can hold the postures or repeat five rounds with the breath.

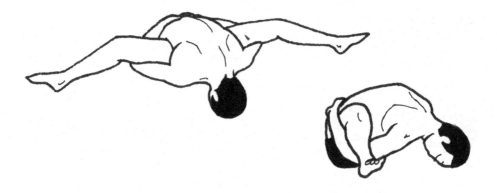

**KURMASANA PARIPURNA** From the above position stretch your arms behind under your thighs to interlock both hands behind. Now open and stretch your legs out to each side as in the side split. Now with the out breath come forward to place your chest and chin on the floor or as close as you can. You can hold the posture and bandhas or repeat it five times with the breath. This variation has a significant role in postures for *Kundalini* awakening. This can benefit young children to be more attentive and controlled with their limbs and mental and emotional behaviour.

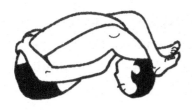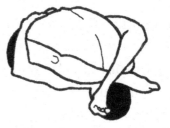

**KURMASANA SAMPURNA** - From the above position keeping your chin to the floor, use your hands and bring your right foot over your head and lock the leg behind the neck, Now bring the left leg over the right and lock it over too. Place your hands behind under your thighs and interlock them behind. Now hold moola bandha with the breath held out therby locking the uddiyana bandha and in this position your jalandhara bandha is naturally held also. This one of the advanced postures in *Kundalini* awakening Yoga postures in Tantra Yoga. The shape of the body becomes like a Kachhap (Kurma) (tortoise), hence the name is *Kurmasana*.

## 28 NIRALAMB PASCHIMOTTANASANA or VAJROLIMUDRA

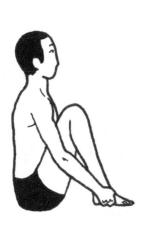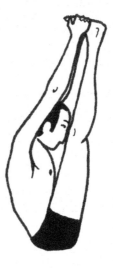

**PROCESS** In *Niralamb Paschimottanasana*, sit on the ground, bend your legs at the knees and hold your ankle joints or toes. Now with the out breath stretch your legs over, balancing on your tailbone and keeping the spine straight, bring your head to your knees. You can hold the posture while holding your breath out or return back with the out breath and repeat five times. You can also hold *Mahabandha* while holding the posture and breath out, which is known as *Vajroli mudra*.

**BENEFITS**
- This asana helps master the body, mind and *prana* and re-establishes harmony as it should be.
- It prevents and can help curing diabetes, heart and blood circulation problems.
- It destroys unnecessary fat and restores a healthy body.
- It is beneficial for backache, tightness in the legs, thighs and hips.
- It is beneficial for men and women in sexual disorders and maintaining celibacy. It strengthens the kidneys.
- It is removes physical and mental lethargy, nervous weakness and enhances the memory.
- It is one of the important practises in *Kundalini* yoga and higher practises to prepare body, mind and *naris* for higher practises and refine *prana*.

CAUTION Persons suffering from ulcer, asthma, tuberculosis of bones, lower back problems, or hip injuries should perform it in a modified way under the supervision of an expert.

DURATION Start with a few seconds, eventually this asana should be performed for two minutes or more for more benefits.

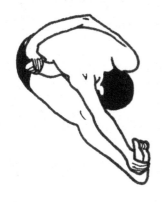 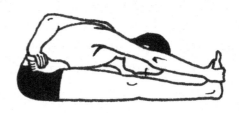

**PROCESS** Sit up straight with legs stretched straight in front on the floor. Bend the left leg at the knee and put it on the right thigh, touching the pelvic area over the genitals. Bring the left hand behind the back and hold the toes of the left foot. Lift up your right arm over your head with the in breath. With the out breath, stretch forward to come down and hold the toes of your right foot with your right hand and gradually place your chest and chin down on your leg. Lift back up with the in breath and repeat the same on the other side.

**SPECIAL** *Ardha* means half, *baddha* means bound, and 'padam' means lotus. This means 'half bound lotus'; and *Paschimottanasana* means stretching from your back to front. So it means 'half-bound-lotus back to front stretch'.

**BENEFITS**
- It activates the kidneys, adrenal glands and pelvic organs.
- It is beneficial in digestive problems, sugar and diabetes.
- It is beneficial for enlarged testicles, hernia and pelvic muscle strength.
- It is a good stretch for the spine, backbone, nervous system and naris.
- It can be practised with *Mahabandha* for *Kundalini* awakening.

**CAUTION** People with dislocated ankle joints, hips or backbone problems should perform this asana carefully under guidance in a modified way such as using a cushion under the knee.

**DURATION** Starting from a few seconds, eventually perform this asana for three minutes for better results.

## 30 GOMUKHASANA

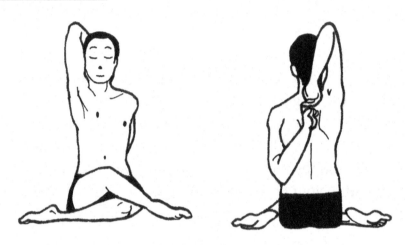

**PROCESS** Sit up straight keeping both the legs straight in front of you. Bend your left leg from the knee and place your foot under the left thigh or buttock. Now bend the right leg and bring your knee on top of the left knee with your right foot placed on the floor close to left buttock. Bring your left hand behind your head and shoulders and then bend the hand from the elbow with the elbow tucked behind over your head and hand hanging down behind the back. Bring your right hand behind from below to reach back to hold the left hand, keeping your right elbow tucked behind your back and waist. Likewise, repeat this with changed legs and hands.

- This asana eliminates backache, stiffness of the shoulders and disorders of the muscles associated with the waist, connecting to shoulders, hips, thighs and back.
- It removes disorders related to the reproductive organs and lungs.
- It brings flexibility to most parts of the body, cleanses and balances prana and the naris, establishing health, vitality, radiance and lightness.

CAUTION This asana should be performed carefully under guidance of Yoga expert if there is any fracture in the bones of the hands, shoulders, thighs and feet.

## 31 BHAIRAVASANA

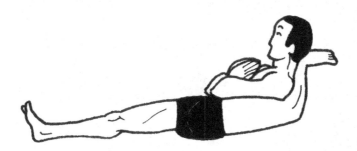

PROCESS Sit up on your Yoga mat. Bring your left leg behind and place your foot behind your neck. Now slowly come up to a standing position on your right leg and join hands into *Namaskar Mudra* to heart. Repeat the same with switched legs.

NOTE 'Bhairav' is a folk Hindu deity. He is remembered with the 64 yoginis or siddhis. In Tantra Yoga, this asana is recognised as a fearsome one. This asana plays a significant role in maintaining concentration and balance.

**BENEFITS**

- This asana is beneficial in preventing and curing diseases related to the kidneys, spleen, the intestines, and adrenal glands.
- This asana increases the digestive capacity.
- It helps improving mental, emotional and physical balance and increases memory.
- It cures and prevents arthritis and joint pain of the knees, hips, shoulders and neck.

**CAUTION** This asana should be performed after attaining perfection in *Hanumanasana* and *Dwipad-Shirasana*.

**DURATION** Perform this asana for three minutes on both legs.

## 32 DWIPADSHIRASANA

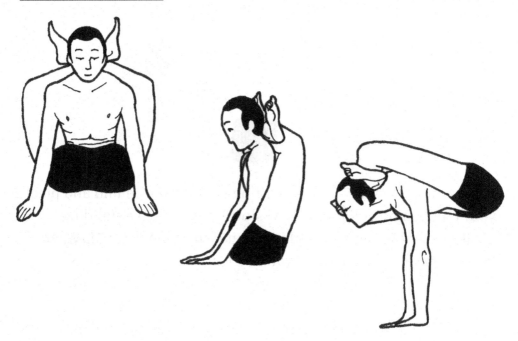

**PROCESS** Place your right foot behind your neck and head and then place your left foot behind, over the right. Now place both your hands firmly on the floor infront and slowly lift and balance on straight arms. Repeat the same with switched sides. Hold *Moolabandha* while you holding your posture.

**NOTE** The word 'Dwipada' means two feet, Sirasa means head and asana means posture. By joining both the feet and head it becomes 'the asana of both feet and head *Dwipadasirasana*.

**BENEFITS**
- Regular performance of this asana provides good massage to the abdomen so it increases digestive capacity.
- It removes disorders related to the uterus, ovaries and gonads.
- It prevents and cures diseases of related to the kidneys, spleen, intestine, and genitals.

**CAUTION** Those who have dislocated joints and scarcity of calcium or weak bones should not perform this asana.

**DURATION** Begin for a few seconds. This asana should be performed for three minutes.

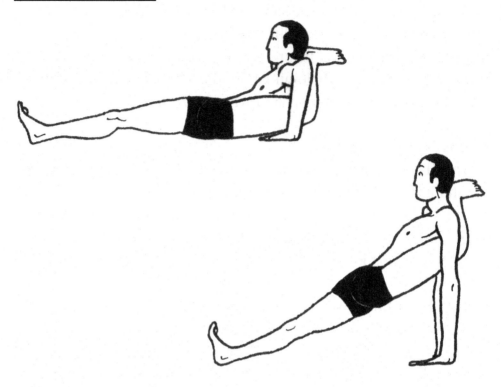

**PROCESS** From a sitting position place your left foot behind your neck and place both your hands on the floor firmly keeping the right leg in front. Now slowly lift and balance up on your straight arms. Likewise, repeat the same with switched legs. Gaze on the tip of your nose while in the posture, holding *Moolabandha*.

**BENEFITS**

- This asana eliminates toxins accumulated in the liver, kidneys, spleen, and stomach. It increases digestive and pelvic health.
- This asana is beneficial for men and women suffering from reproductive issues.
- This asana is beneficial for the joints of shoulders, back and hips.

**CAUTION** Persons with weak elbows, shoulders, and arms should perform this asana carefully, under guidance.

## 34 BRAHMCHARYASANA

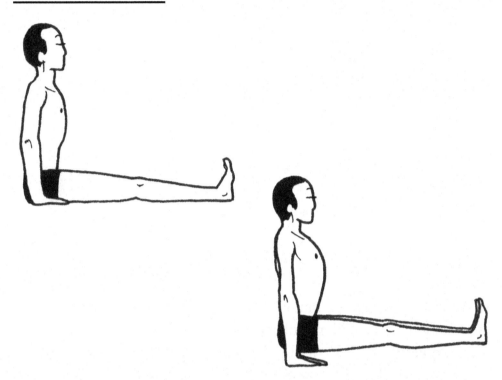

**PROCESS** Sit up straight with legs stretched in front and keep them together. Place both your hands on the floor close to your hips and slowly lift the legs and buttocks up and balance on your straight hands. Hold the posture while holding *Moolabandha*.

**BENEFITS**
- This asana is really helpful in maintaining celibacy and redirects sexual energy to a higher energy.
- The joints shoulders, elbows and hips become strong and flexible.
- Stimulates and strengthen abdominal and pelvic organs and muscles.
- It brings vitality, strength and balance and increases memory and the power of concentration.
- It stimulates all the body charkas and awakens the Kundalini.

## 35 ASTAVAKRASANA

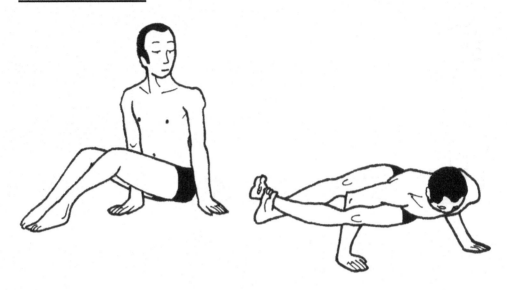

**PROCESS** Sit on your Yoga mat with your knees bent and place your right hand firmly in the middle of both legs close to your thigh and your left hand out side over the left thigh. Now slowly lift up and balance your whole body on slightly bent elbows with the legs pointing out to the right side.

**SPECIAL** In this asana eight joints, wrists, elbows, ankles, knees, hips, waist, back and neck are tilted or bent and is hence known as *Asta-Vakra-Asana* (Eight-tilted-pose ).

There was a saint known as Aastavakra, whose eight parts of the body were crooked from his birth and he was 'de-formed'. He was the spiritual guru of Raja Janaka, the king of Mithila. Aastavakra defeated Acharya Dandi in philosophical debate, in the court of Raja Janaka. He took the revenge of the defeat of his father Kahol, and achieved a respectful and dignified position. It is said that when the saint was in his mother's womb, he heard his father uttering Veda mantras incorrectly and made a mockery of it. The father cursed him and, therefore, he got the shape of Aastavakra. This asana is dedicated to him.

- This asana stimulates and strengthens by putting pressure on the digestive system , giving it a good massage. Essential secretions of liver, spleen, pancreas and stomach are balanced and digestive capacity, body immunity and vitality are increased.
- This asana can prevent hernias and reduces fat around the abdomen, hips and pelvis.
- This asana stimulates the nervous system and brings harmony and peace.
- Helps strengthening shoulders, arms and pelvic muscles.

**CAUTION** Perform this asana along with *Titibhasana* and *Bakasana*. Those who have dislocated joints and fractured bones, weak elbows and knees should perform this asana under strict guidance.

**DURATION** This asana should be mastered for three minutes.

## 36 AAKARN DHANURASANA

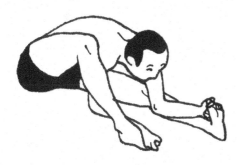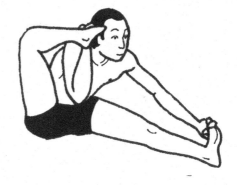

**PROCESS** Sit with your legs straight in front. Bend your right leg from the knee and hold your big toe with the right hand and also hold the big toe of left foot with the left hand. Now with your in breath pull your right leg towards your head and touch your toes to your ears, while keeping the left leg straight. Gaze at the left foot. Repeat the same with switched legs and hands.

**SPECIAL** When the archer aims for his target, he pulls the cord of the bow to the ear for force and speed, so the arrow reaches the target. The posture of this asana resembles this and therefore. It is known as *Aakarn* (up to the ear) *Dhanurasana* (bow posture).

**BENEFITS**
- This asana removes stiffness and toxins and prevents and cures pain in all the joints of the body.
- It broadens the chest and opens the heart and shoulders.
- It strengthens the lungs and heart.
- It stimulates and strengthens the digestive system pelvic organs.
- It is especially helpful in the treatment of liver and spleen diseases.

**CAUTION** Patients suffering from asthma, tuberculosis or a weak backbone should practise this asana in the presence of a Yoga expert.

**DURATION** For better results, perform this asana for three minutes with *Moolabandha* and *Bddiyana bandha*.

## 37 GARBHASANA

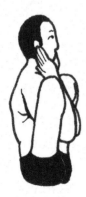 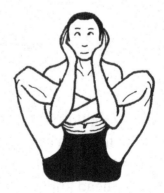

**PROCESS** Sit straight in *Padmasana*. Put both the hands through the gap between your legs and thighs inside the knees, as in *Kukuttasana*, pull them upwards to hold your ears. Maintaining your balance on your sitting bones, gaze in the middle of your eye brows.

**SPECIAL** In this asana, the shape of the body resembles an embryo in the womb, and hence is known as *Gargha-asana* (embryo or foetus-posture). This asana belongs to the family of '*Padmasana*' like *Baddhpadmasana*, *Yogmudrasana* and *Kukuttasana*. This asana affects the whole body. It should be performed after achieving good practise of *Kukuttasana*.

**BENEFITS**
- This asana strengthens the lungs, heart, abdominal and pelvic organs by giving them a good massage.
- It refines the blood, naris and prana and can prevent and cure skin diseases, blood disorders, thyroid and reproductive disorders.
- The Sciatic nerves are relieved, stimulated and strengthened.
- It brings physical, mental and emotional stability and cures lethargy, heaviness or lack of interest.

**CAUTION** Person with dislocated joints and fractured bones should perform this asana under the guidance of a Yoga expert.

**DURATION** Begin it for a few seconds and then master for three minutes or more with *Moolabandha*.

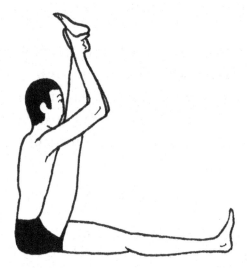

**PROCESS** Sit up straight and raise your right leg straight high as much as possible. Catch your ankle and try to touch the chin to the knee without folding the leg. This is the *Stambhan asana*. Slowly release the pose and repeat the same with the left leg.

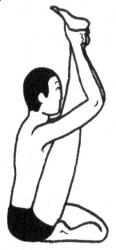

**STAMBHAM ASANA SAPURN** Sit straight in a cross legged position with the right leg on top. Now hold your right foot with both hands and slowly stretch your leg straight in front of the chest with the in breath and return back the with out breath. Repeat the same with the left leg.

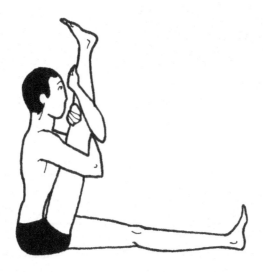

**SATAMBHAMA ASANA SAMPURNA** Sit straight and come to *Stambhama asana* with the right leg. Now wrap your arms around your right thigh with foot over your head and leg straight. Try to breath out fully with *Mukha-bhastrika*, hold your breath out while holding *Mahabandha*.

**BENEFITS**

- It helps stimulate and strengthen the hips, knees, and lower back joints and all the associated muscles.
- This series of asana stimulates kidneys, adrenal glands, reproductive organs and abdominal organs and prevents and cures all the associated problems of these areas.
- This asana refines naris and blood and reactivates the nervous system, increasing health and vitality.
- This series helps cure lethargy, heaviness, un-attentiveness, mental and emotional instability, and other mental and emotional disorders.
- This asana helps in gross or lower energies to higher energies and awakens *Kundalini*.

**DURATION** You can practise the series from three to five minutes for desired benefits.

## 39 BADDHA KONA ASANA

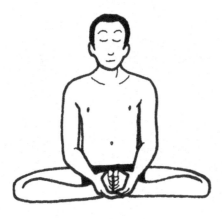 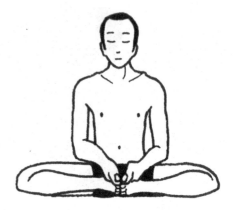

Sit straight while keeping both the legs straight in front. Slowly fold the legs and place sole against sole firmly. If possible place your heels against the groin firmly. Hold the big toes with the index finger and thumb firmly. Sit straight with the erect spine.

**BADDHA KONA ASANA MUDRAS** You can practise following mudras for energy work on various chakras as well as stimulating various parts of your brain:

- Hold the big toes with the index fingers and thumbs.
- Clasp both hands together around both feet together.

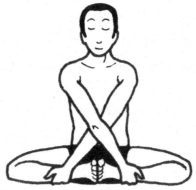

- Hold to your legs with crossed arms, holding the left leg with the right hand and right leg with left hand.

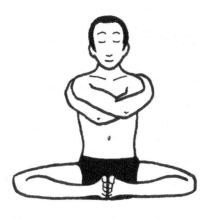 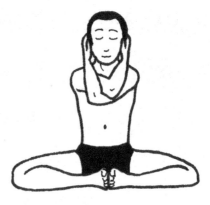

- Cross your hands across the chest and place your palms on shoulders.
- Cross your hands and hold to your ears.

**BENEFITS**

- In this asana the body comes into a beautiful triangle energy bounded position. This is of great importance for spiritual development.
- This asana has great importance in tantric practises of *Kundalini* awakening.
- It is very good for the brain, and nervous system. It helps in aligning the hip area and hip joints.
- It also stimulates the inner thighs and keeps them flexible.
- It encourages proper blood circulation in the pelvic region, thighs and the genital organs and thus prevents development of cancers in this area due to the psychic type of cleansing that can occur through the practices.
- *Baddha Kona asana* practice also has great importance for women during pregnancy and for those who are planning to have a child.
- It will also help in the safe and easy delivery of a healthy child.
- This asana is extremely good for the sex glands and the hip joints and it is very helpful for those experiencing premature ejaculations other sexual problems and menstrual disorders, etc.

## 40 PRATIPAHALASANA

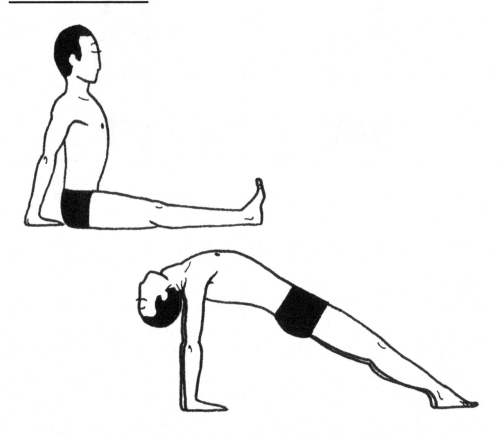

**PROCESS** Sit straight with your legs stretched in front. Place both your hands behind your body with fingers facing towards the buttocks. Slowly lift your body up on your straight hands and stretch your legs out to touch your toes to the floor. Hold your posture for few breaths.

**BENEFITS** This is one of the closing postures and helps lift the energy from the lower to higher energy centres and helps you to follow visualisations and *Jnana-Yoga kriyas* during relaxation. It strengthens the shoulders and arms and opens the chest.

## CHAPTER 5

# ASANA PRACTICES AND SEQUENCES FROM CROSS LEGGED

## 41 YOGAMUDRASANA

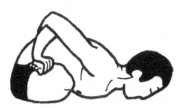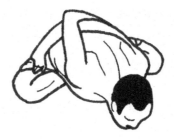

Come to *Baddhpadmasana*. Now take a deep in breath. While slowly breathing out, bend forward from your hips and waist to place your chin or forehead on the floor, aiming to bring your chest flat to the floor. You can return back to an upright seated position with the in breath, or hold the posture as long as you can hold your breath out while holding *Mahabandha*. Likewise, touch your chin or forehead to the ground over the left knee to the left side while exhaling. Withdraw from the asana gradually while inhaling the breath and repeat to the right side.

**SPECIAL** This is a special posture of Yoga as it includes asana and mudras. This is called *Yogamudrasana* because in *Baddhpadmasana*, the head is bowed down and the nose touches the ground (a gesture of gratitude and salutation). This asana is considered very important for awakening the *Kundalini*, transcending lower energy to higher.

**BENEFITS**
- It provides a good stretch for the abdominal and pelvic muscles, thus stimulating and activating the abdominal and pelvic organs.
- It refines gross energies to subtle energies and brings lightness, vitality and radiance.
- It balances the left and right sides or masculine-feminine energies and the autonomic nervous system, resulting in a

balanced and stable personality.
- It cures diseases such as constipation, indigestion, infertility, arthritis, lethargy, and muscular weakness.
- This asana prevents and cures problems of kidneys and spleen and makes them strong.

**CAUTION** This asana should be performed under strict guidance in a modified way if there are chronic or serious problems with backbone, hips, or shoulders.

**DURATION** This asana can be performed as three to five rounds on each side, or from a few seconds up to three minutes as a full series.

### YOGAMUDRASANA VARIATIONS

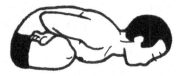

**HAND VARIATION 1** Place the left hand at the navel and the right hand on top of the left and perform *Yogamudrasana.*

**HAND VARIATION 2** Close both fists, keeping thumbs closed tight inside and join the hands together under the navel and perform *Yogamudrasana.*

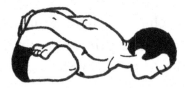

**HAND VARIATION 3** Hold both hands behind your back and perform *Yogamudrasana.*

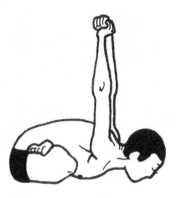

**HAND VARIATION 4** Interlock the hands behind your back and as you perform *Yogamudrasana* also stretch your arms up behind your back, aiming to bring them straight over your shoulders.

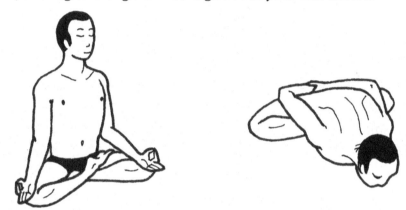

**YOGAMUDRASANA SAPURN** Perform *Yogamudrasana* with different hand variations in *Sukhasana* or a cross-legged position.

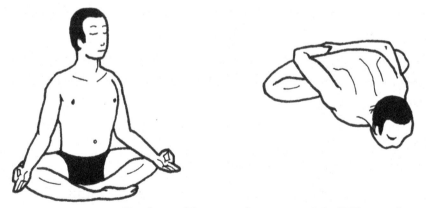

**YOGAMUDRASANA APURN** Perform *Yogamudrasana* with different hand variations in *Ardha-Padmasana*.

## 42 PARVATASANA

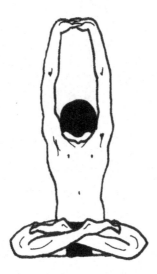

**PROCESS** 'Parvat' means mountain. Our body takes the shape of a mountain in this asana. Sit straight in *Padmasana* (if you cannot perform *Padmasana* then choose *Sukhasana, Ardhapadmasana,* or *Siddhasana*) and interlock the fingers of both hands over your head. Now stretch your hands up over your head as high as you can. Bring your chin down and place it against your chest in *Jalandhara bandha*. Hold the posture from a few seconds to a minute. You can also use *Anjali mudra* instead of interlocked hands.

**BENEFITS**
- This asana removes stiffness of the shoulders, arms and elbows and prevents and relieves arthritis and gout.
- It widens the chest and shoulders and opens the lungs and heart.
- It re-aligns and activates the chakras and transcends our energy from lower to higher.
- It is good for the joints and associated muscles of the knees, thighs, ankles, backbone and shoulders.

**SPECIAL** This asana brings strength, stability and grounding as the mountains on our mother earth standing and nurturing in each and every weather situation.

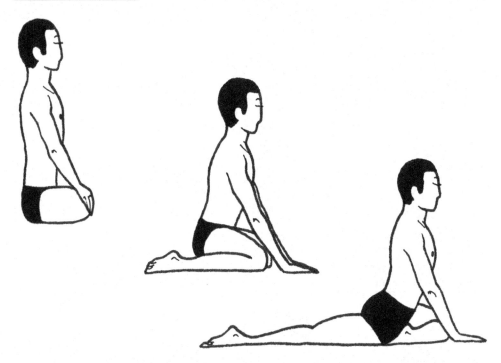

**PROCESS** Come to *Sukhasana* and place your hands on the floor in front for support. Now slowly stretch your right leg backward as straight as you can while keeping the left foot tucked against the genitals.

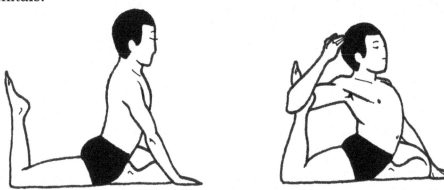

Now bend your right leg from your knee, pointing your foot up to the ceiling. Bring your right hand behind and hold the right foot in your inner elbow and let your hand point back towards the head.

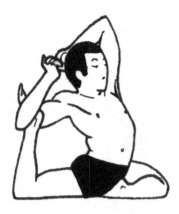

Slowly lift your left hand over your head to reach back to hold to the right hand, with your elbow pointing over your head. Return back to *Sukhasana* and practise on the other side.

**RAJKAPOTASANA VARIATIONS**

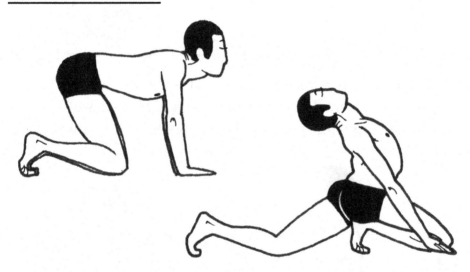

**RAJKAPOTASANA PURNA** Come to *Chatuspadasana*. Now slowly bring your right leg forward with the knee, leg and foot flat on the floor in the middle of both hands. Gently push your left leg straight back and sit straight on the right foot with hands to both sides of your knee on the floor. Look upward and bend back, creating a beautiful arch of the head, neck, spine and leg. Return back to *Chatuspadasana* and repeat with changed sides.

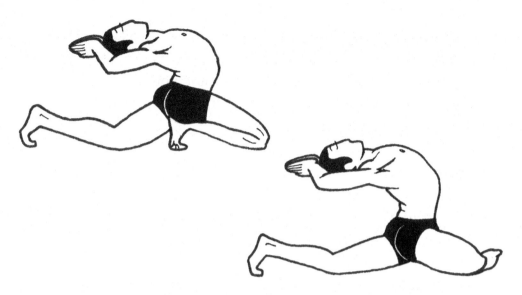

**RAJKAPOTASANA SAPURN** From *Rajkapotasana-Apurn* slowly lift both hands over your head and join together in *Anjali mudra* and bend back as much as you can. Repeat with both sides.

**RAJKAPOTASANA PURNA** From *Chatuspadasana* slowly bring your right knee forward with the knee going across to the right hand and foot to the left hand. Slowly push your left leg back aiming to place your buttocks on the floor. Slowly lift your right hand over your head and stretch back with support of the left hand from front. You can also try to lift both hands over in *Anjali mudra* and stretch back. Come back to chatuspadasana and repeat with changed sides.

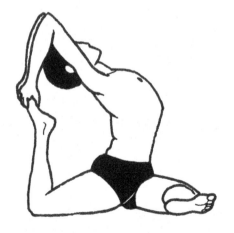
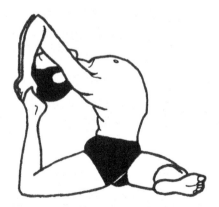

**RAJKAPOTASANA PARIPURNA** Come to *Rajkapotasana* purn as above and bend your right leg at the back from your knee. Slowly lift both hands over your head and reach back to hold your foot with both hands. Your elbows should be pointing up over your head. Repeat the same with left leg at back.

**RAJKAPOTASANA SAMPURN** From *Rajakapotasana Paripurna* try to bend further back as well as bringing your foot towards your head to reach back to place your head on your right foot. Hold your foot with both hands with elbows pointing over your head.

**SPECIAL** The word 'Rajkapot' means king of pigeons. This asana is attractive and beautiful, with the chest brought forward and opening wide, it is given the name '*Rajkapotasana*'.

**BENEFITS**
- This asana is beneficial for the shoulders, arms, chest, back, hips, knees and legs. It's a complete work out for your body from toes to head and stretches almost each muscles throughout the body.
- This asana is beneficial for digestive system, pelvic organs and reproductive organs.
- This asana eliminates the toxins accumulated in the joints and muscles in our body and brings health, vitality and lightness.
- This asana series cures mental and emotional disorders, lethargy and lack of interest.

**CAUTION** Persons suffering from sciatica, hip injuries or shoulder injuries should perform this series under guidance in a modified way.

## 44 GUPT PADMASANA

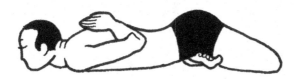

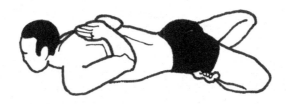

**PROCESS** Sit in *Padmasana* and lie down on your front. Now bring your hands behind the back and join them in Namaskar Mudra with fingers pointing towards the head. Hold *Moolabandha* while you holding your posture.

**BENEFITS**
- It makes the spine straight and opens *Sushumna Nari* to be ready for the entry of *Kundalini* energy and for it to travel upwards.
- It widens the chest and opens the shoulders.
- This asana prevents and cures the diseases of the liver and the spleen.
- It eliminates a pain in the shoulders, waist, knees and hips.
- This asana cures skin diseases, blood impurities, dysentery, asthma, cough and migraine.

**CAUTION** This asana should be performed along with *Gomukhasana* and *Padmasana*.

**DURATION** One can hold this posture from a few seconds to three minutes or more to meditate.

## 45 KUKUTTASANA

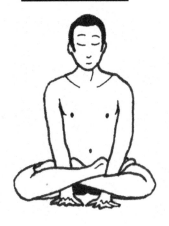 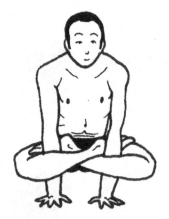 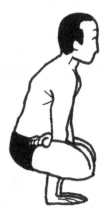

**PROCESS** Sit straight in *Padmasana*. Put both the hands through the folding space of the legs inside the knees and place the palms on the ground. Slowly lift up the whole body and balance on your straight arms.

**NOTE** The yogis invented so many special asanas copying the shapes of animals and birds and achieved the same benefits as the animals derived from these asanas (strength, power, stamina etc). 'Kukutta' is a Sanskrit word that means a cockrel. This asana is called *Kukuttasana* because in this the body resembles a cockrel.

**BENEFITS**
- It strengthens shoulders and arms and the opens the chest and heart area.
- The spinal cord becomes strong, flexible and straight and hence ready for *Kundalini* energy to travel upwards.
- It strengthens abdominal and pelvic muscles and cures or prevents diseases of these areas.
- It cleanses the blood, naris and prana and cures skin diseases, blood disorders, dysentery, asthma, cough and chronic fever.
- It brings lightness and vitality and cures lethargy and weakness of body and mind.

- It helps to keep the mind and body in harmony and balance.

**CAUTION** People who have dislocated joints of the knees, ankles, wrists, elbows and shoulders and broken bones should not perform this asana.

**DURATION** Perform this asana for one to three minutes for the best results.

## CHAPTER 6

# SITTING TWISTS

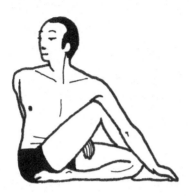

**PROCESS** Sit up on a blanket or a Yoga mat with the legs straight in front. Fold the left leg and place the heel close to the genitals. Then set the sole of the right foot towards the left knee. Bend the right leg, hold onto the foot for support and then place your right foot on the floor over your left knee close to the thigh. Lift your left hand over to place your shoulder over the right knee, gently twisting your arm to reach down to hold to right foot. Now bring your right hand behind your back to place it over left thigh towards navel. Untwist yourself and then repeat the same with changed sides.

**BENEFITS**
- This asana is good for the backbone, neck, arms, shoulders, hips and chest.
- It sends a good message to the abdominal and pelvic organs and stimulates them to function properly.
- It provides flexibility to the backbone and associated muscles from back to waist, hips, pelvis and abdomen.
- It activates the spleen and liver and prevents sugar, diabetes and heart problems.
- It balances the secretion of insulin and eliminates diabetes.

**SPECIAL** This asana is dedicated to Matsyendranath, Great Yogi and master of Hatha Yoga in the Natha tradition. 'Matsyendranath' is also known as Machhindranath. In the '*Hatha Yoga Pradipika*' it is stated that, whilst Shiva was describing the secrets of Yoga to Parvati, his wife on a sea shore, it was also overheard by a fish. When Shiva offered water to the sun and poured it in the sea, the fish assumed a splendid form and became Matsyendranath, and Lord Shiva blessed him to go out in world and teach Yoga to worldly people to be healthy, happy and liberated.

**CAUTION** Those with fractured bones and dislocated joints should perform this asana under guidance in modified variations. Pregnant women must avoid this asana.

**DURATION** This asana series should be performed for a few seconds to three minutes on each side.

## 47 MATSYENDRASANA

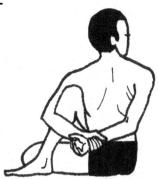

**PROCESS** In this asana, fold the left leg and place the foot on the right thigh close to pelvis. Place the right foot outside the left knee close to the thigh on the floor while keeping your knee upright. Now lift your left arm straight over and place the shoulder over or against the right knee, twisting your arm inward to reach down to hold the right foot with the left hand. Now bring your right hand from behind to point to your navel or over the thigh. Twist over to look over the right shoulder. Untwist and then repeat the same on the other side.

**MATSENDRASANA PARIPURNA** From *Matsendrasana* you can turn your left arm around the left leg over the knee and bring the right hand from behind to reach back and hold both hands together. Repeat the same with changed legs and hands.

**BENEFITS** Along with *Ardhamatsyendrasana*, these series of postures also possess special spiritual benefits. Once you lock your foot against the pelvis and lock your thighs and hips in place with arms and shoulders, it forces all the inner organs against each other providing an amazing massage to organs in the pelvic, abdominal and chest area. This provides a deep stretch and stimulation to the associated muscles and ligaments. It cleanses the naris and allows the vital energy to flow freely.

**CAUTION** Pregnant women must avoid this series of twists as they go deep through the pelvis, womb and supporting organs, which will have adverse effects onthe foetus. Also, if you have injuries or dislocated joints, practise these asanas only under guidance taking a modified and gradual approach.

## 48 MARICHAYA ASANA

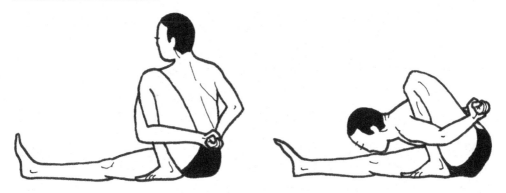

**PROCESS** Sit straight with your legs stretched in front. Fold your right leg while bringing your knee to the shoulder. Stretch your right arm straight in front and curl it around the right leg. Turn and bring your left hand to reach back to hold the right hand behind. Now come forward to place your head on top of the left knee and hold your posture. Repeat the same with changed sides.

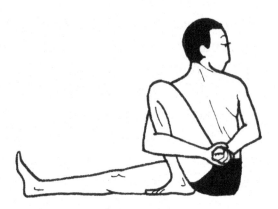

**MARICHAYA ASANA SAPURN** Sit straight with your legs stretched in front. Place your right foot close to the right thigh with the knee pointing up towards to your shoulder. Now stretch over the left leg to bring the right arm forward, and wrap it back around the right leg while reaching behind to hold the right hand with the left hand. Now try to come back up right and turn to left and look behind, twisting the upper chest and shoulder area. Repeat the same on the other side.

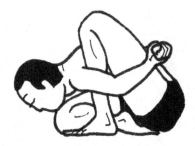

**MARICHAYA ASANA PURNA** Sit straight in *Sukhasana* and then bring your right knee over and behind the right shoulder. Wrap your right arm from the front and left from the back to reach back to hold to your hands and then place your chin on left knee. Repeat the same with changed sides.

**BENEFITS**

- This asana provides a good massage to abdominal and pelvic organs, preventing and curing all the associated problems.
- It's a good twist and opening posture for the upper chest and shoulder area and brings health and vitality in the chest and shoulder areas.
- This series stimulates the spinal nervous system and balances the autonomic nervous system, bringing balance and stability.
- This asana helps align the knees, thigh bones, hips and lower back and prepares the body and mind for *Kundalini* awakening.

**DURATION** One should practise this asana from a few seconds to three minutes for desired benefits.

## CHAPTER 7

# ASANA PRACTICES AND SEQUENCES FROM FOUR FOOTED

## 49 TITIBHASANA

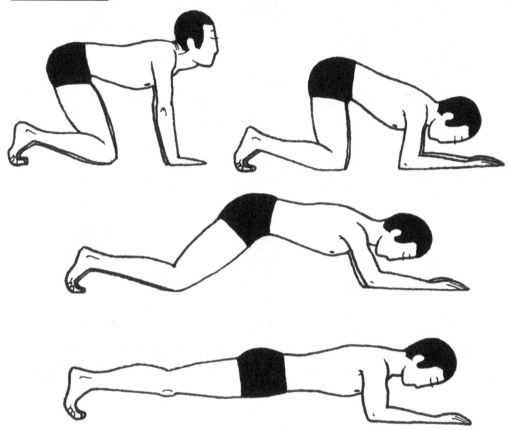

**PROCESS** Come to *Chatuspadasana* and place your elbows on the floor under your shoulders and palms on the floor firmly infront. Slowly step your knees back, tuck your toes in on the floor, lift your knees up and stretch up straight from the heels to head, balancing on your elbows and toes.

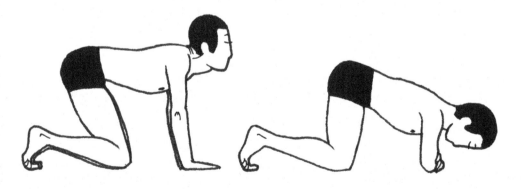

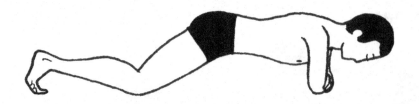

**TITIBHASANA SAPURNA** As above come to *Chatus-padasana* and place your elbows on the floor under your shoulders, crossing your lower arms to hold to your elbows. Now step your knees back as far as you can and try to hold your spine and head in a straight line.

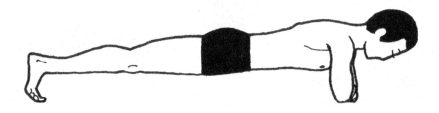

**TITIBHASANA PURNA** As above with arms crossed under shoulders, step your legs back and balance straight on your toes and crossed arms.

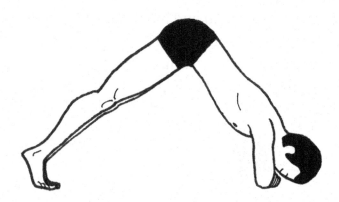

**TITBHASANA SAMPURNA** As above, once you can balance on your elbows and toes, slowly walk your toes forward, lifting up your buttocks as high as you can. Your body takes a sloping mountain position and let your head stay close to your arms.

**BENEFITS**

- This asana improves and strengthens arms, shoulders, spinal and pelvic muscles.
- It removes the toxins and stiffness from elbows, shoulders, back, knees and ankles and they become strong and flexible.
- This asana is good to prepare for a healthy conception and pregnancy. However, this asana should not be performed during pregnancy.
- This asana is beneficial for liver, and pancreas.
- This asana brings our body back to a healthy shape.

**CAUTION** If you have any serious problems in your shoulders, elbows and spinal joints perform this asana under guidance in modified way.

## CHAPTER 8

# ASANA PRACTICES AND SEQUENCES FROM FACE PRONE

## 50 DHANURASANA

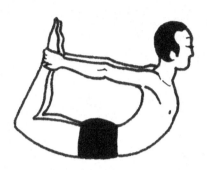 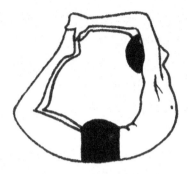

**PROCESS:** Lie flat on your front. Fold both the legs from the knees upward and reach back with both hands to hold your feet. Pull the feet with full power while inhaling to lift your legs, knees, chest and head up as far as you can go, arching the back. You can aim to finally balance on your navel. Pull the neck up. Your back and waist will automatically bend in a bow shape. The body assumes the shape of a Dhanush (bow), hence the posture is known as *Dhanurasana*. Return back from the asana slowly while exhaling the breath. Since this asana involves more strength, it should be followed by *Shavasana* and relaxation.

### BENEFITS

- It strengthens the muscles of the arms, chest, waist, legs and abdomen and widens the chest.
- The backbone becomes supple and strong.
- Toxins and stiffness accumulated in the areas of shoulders, knees, ankles, thighs, hips and wrists are eliminated, and these parts become flexible and strong.
- This is a good stretch for the abdomen and pelvis and so helps to prevent and cure problems such as weak appetite, constipation, indigestion; increased fat and intestinal gas problems, weak pelvic and core muscles, and infertility.
- This helps to open the heart and lung area.

- This is helpful in increasing height in children.
- This helps in maintaining normal and healthy blood circulation.
- It cleanses naris and refines our energy into subtle prana, refreshing and rejuvenating the whole body, mind and soul, leading to health and vitality.
- This full series is beneficial and recommended for young children.

**CAUTION** Those who are suffering from hernia, ulcer, chronic back problems, dislocated joints or fractures or with intestinal disorders should perform this asana only under strict guidance in a modified way.

**DURATION** Begin by practicing it for a few rounds and gradually build up the strength to hold the posture from 30 seconds to three minutes, or practise the whole series for five minutes or more.

**DHANURASANA VARIATIONS**

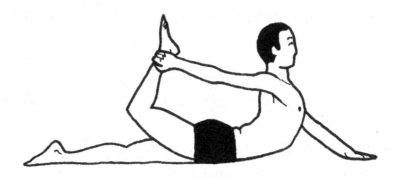

**DHANURASANA EKA PADA SAPURNA** From the front lying position bring your left hand on the floor over your chest and reach back with the right hand to hold on to the right foot. Now with the in breath, pull and lift up your right leg, head and chest using your left hand on the floor for support. This is a modified variation if you cannot do the full posture.

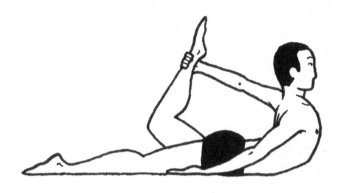

**DHANURASANA EKA PADA PURNA** Lie down straight on your front with both arms stretched down along the legs. Bend your right leg and hold your leg, or ankle joint or foot with right hand. With the in breath, pull and lift up your leg, chest and head up as far as you can. Return back with the out breath. Repeat the same on the left side. You can repeat five rounds on each side or hold your posture from 30 seconds to one minute.

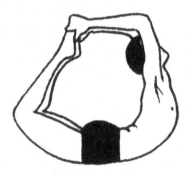

**DHANURASANA SAPURNA** From the front lying position bend both legs and reach back to hold to both legs, ankle joints or feet. Now with the in breath lift your legs, chest and head upward while pulling your legs upward. Return back with the out breath. You can repeat this five times with the breath, gradually building up the strength to hold your posture from 30 seconds to three minutes.

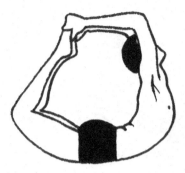 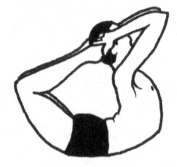

**DHANURASANA PURNA** Repeat the same as above while holding your big toes with index fingers and thumbs. You can try to lift and stretch up as far as possible, gradually building up to completely balancing on the navel. You can repeat with the breath or hold the posture to your comfort.

**DHANURASANA PARIPURNA** As above, holding the big toes with the index fingers, now lift your head, chest and legs and stretch while pulling your toes to your ears. Gradually build up to touch the toes to both ears. In the beginning repeat it 5 times moving into the posture on the in breath releasing on the out breath, then gradually work towards holding the posture and gradually work towards holding the posture.

**DHANURASANA SAMPURNA** Holding your feet over the toes, lift and stretch over as high as you can, gradually aiming to balance on your navel with feet and hands coming straight over the navel in the stretch. Hold *Mulabandha* as long as you can hold the posture.

**SPECIAL** This whole series is amazingly beneficial for children to build strength, flexibility, endurance and attentiveness.

## 51 BHUJANGASANA

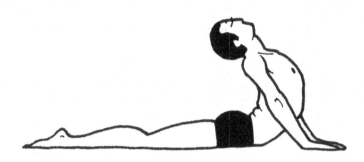

**PROCESS** Lie down on your front; keep the knees, ankles, heels, and feet together. Place both your hands on the floor, with your palms at the shoulders. With the in breath lift up your head and chest using your hands for support, straightening the arms. You can lift up to your navel creating a nice back curve of the spine. Slowly release with the out breath. You can hold the posture from 30 seconds to three minutes.

### BENEFITS
- This asana helps the spinal vertebra to be flexible and strong, widens the chest, opens the shoulders and lengthens the arm muscles. This asana if practised carefully can help with dislocated vertebra and back pain.
- It shapes men and women around the chest and shoulders.
- It removes constipation and corrects the blood circulation.
- It strengthens the digestive system.
- It stimulates spinal nerves and increases concentration and memory .
- Those who wish to increase their height must perform this asana.

**SPECIAL** The posture of this asana is like a hooded cobra. Therefore it is called *Bhujangasana* or *Sarpasana*. In the beginning, one faces many difficulties in performing this asana but it becomes easy with regular exercise. According to yogis, this asana is helpful in awakening the *Kundalini*.

**CAUTION** Patients suffering from tuberculosis, chronic back pain, shoulder dislocation or ulcers should perform this asana under supervision in a modified way.

**DURATION** Perform this asana series for two to five minutes for better results.

**BHUJANGASANA VARIATIONS**

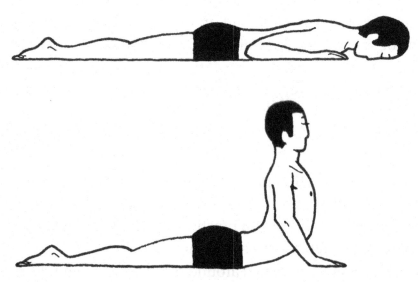

**BHUJANGASANA KRIYA 1** Lie down straight on your front, and place both your hands close to your shoulders with the elbows close to the waist. With the in breath lift your head and chest up as far as you can without taking any support from the hands and arms. Gently hiss your breath out to return back to the floor. Repeat three or five times.

**BHUJANGASANA KRIYA 2** As above, this time with the in breath push up with your hands to stretch back as far as you can and release back down hissing your breath out. Repeat three to five times.

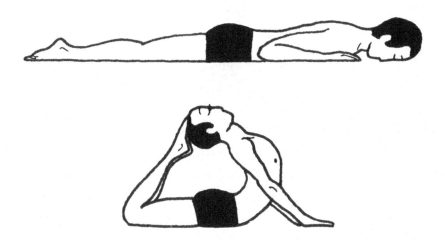

**BHUJANGASANA KRIYA 3** As above, this time with the in breath as you lift your chest and head up into *Bhujangasana,* also bend your legs at the knees aiming to touch your feet to your head. Return back with hissing your breath out. Repeat three to five times.

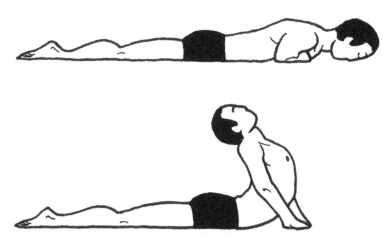

**BHUJANGASANA KRIYA 4** From a front lying position place both your hands under the upper chest with the fingers interlaced. With the in breath push and lift up your head, shoulders and chest up to the navel. Return back with hissing your breath out. Repeat three to five rounds.

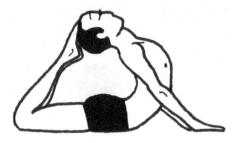

**BHUJANGASANA PURNA** From a front lying position with your hands on the floor close to yours shoulders, with the in breath push on your arms to lift your head, chest and shoulders up to come to *Bhujangasana*. Take a few deep breaths and then gently bend your legs at the knees to bring your feet over and touch your head. Hold your posture from 10 seconds to one minute.

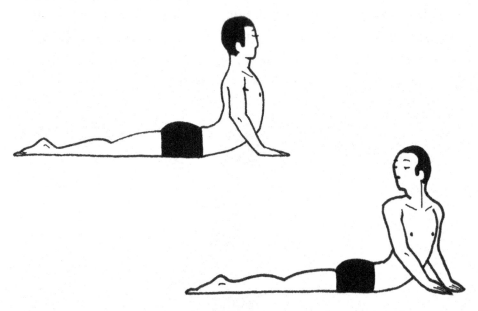

**BHUJANGASANA TIRIYAKA** From *Bhujangasana,* with the in breath, turn your head, shoulders and chest around to right side and gaze back at your heels. Return back with the out breath and repeat the same on the left side.

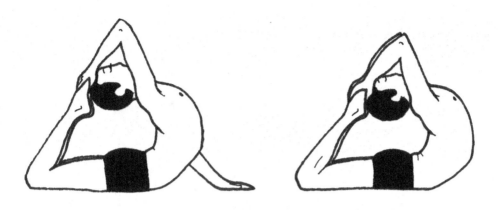

**BHUJANGASANA SAMPURNA** Come to *Bhujangasana-Purna* and hold it for 30 seconds. Now gently lift one hand up to reach back to hold your toes and gradually bring your other hand up to hold the other foot. Here your elbows are pointing over your head and face. You can hold the posture from 10 seconds to one minute.

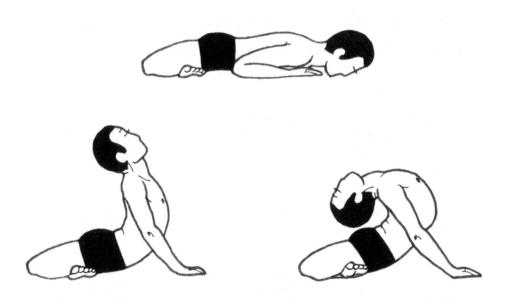

**BHUJANGASANA PADMA** Come to *Padmasana* and lie down on your front. Now practise *Bhujangasana* as you were doing with straight legs. One can aim to touch the buttocks with the head. You can hold the posture from 10 seconds to one minute.

## 52 SHALBHASANA

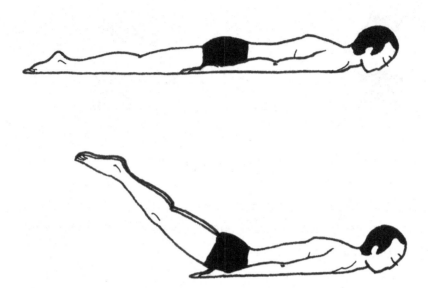

**PROCESS** Lie down straight on your front. Place both hands beneath the thighs for support. You can keep the palms upward or close your fists under. Lift up both the legs up as far as you can while keeping legs together and straight.

### SHALBHASANA VARIATIONS

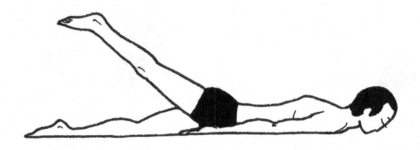

**SHALBHASANA EKAPADA** As above lift right leg up with in breath and hold for few breaths. Repeat the same with the left leg.

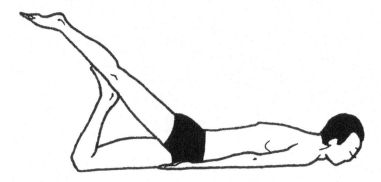

**SHALBHASANA EKAPADA SALAMBA** From a front lying position bend your left leg from the knee with the foot pointing up to the ceiling. Now lift your right leg up and place your knee on top of the left foot and push up as far as you can go. Repeat the same with the opposite leg.

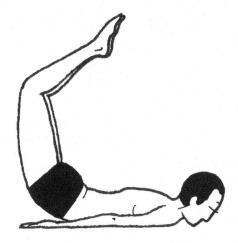

**SHALBHASANA SALAMBA** Lie down on your front with the legs up against a wall and start pushing your legs over to the wall as in *Shalbhasana*, as far as you can go. This will help to prepare you for some of the advance variations.

**SHALBHASANA PURNA** In a front lying position while keeping your hands under the thighs, bend both the knees and point your feet up. Try to lift and jerk your knees up as if you are going to place them on top of your head. Hold your posture on the chest and abdominal area, with the spine and legs forming a nice arching curve.

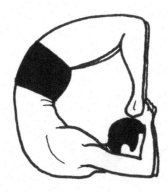

**SHALBHASANA PARIPURNA** As in *Shalbhasana Purna* now slowly bring your feet or toes on top of your head and hold your posture.

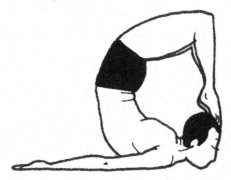

**SHALBHASANA NIRALAMBA** Come to *Shalbhasana Paripurna* and slowly bring your hands over your head to hold to your feet.

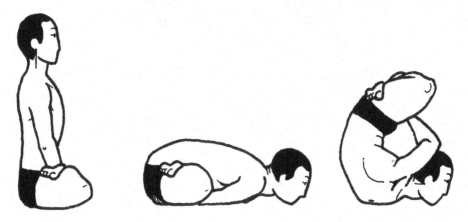

**SHALBHASANA PADAM** Sit up straight in *Padmasana* and slowly lie on your front in *Padmasana*. Using your hands under your thighs draw your knees over your head in Padamasna and hold your posture.

- This asana prevents diabetes, heart disease and nervous disorders.
- It stimulates digestive secretions and increases appetite, removes indigestion and constipation.
- It makes the chest wide and the waist strong.
- It makes the backbone flexible, stimulates the nervous system and eliminates fatigue.
- It shapes the body and encourages all the organs into their correct positions.
- It increases attentiveness, concentration and memory.
- It prevents and cures diseases like sinus, cough, fever and weakness.
- This series is important in *Kundalini* awakening and *Nari Suddhi* or cleansing.

**CAUTION** Those who have ulcers, tuberculosis, tuberculosis of bones, dislocated joints or fractured bones should perform this asana series under guidance.

**DURATION** Perform this asana series for five minutes or more for better results.

## 53  VIPREET PASCHIMOTTASANA

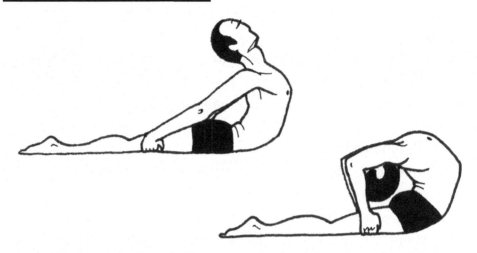

**PROCESS** Lie on your front. Lift up your head, chest and shoulders as in *Bhujangasana* while reaching back with the hands to hold your legs or ankle joints. Gradually aim to bring your head behind you to touch your buttocks.

### BENEFITS

- This is an extreme back bend and leads to strength, flexibility and endurance of the back bone.
- It prevents and cures kidney, bladder, uterus and genital disorders.
- It cleanses the naris and opens *Sushumna* nari for *Kundalini* energy to travel upward.
- It prevents diabetes and heart diseases.
- It regulates the blood circulation.

**CAUTION** Those who are suffering from tuberculosis-infected bones, chronic back problems, ulcer, hypertension, and hypotension should perform this asana under guidance.

**DURATION** This asana brings good results even if practised from a few seconds to thirty seconds.

# INVERTED POSTURES

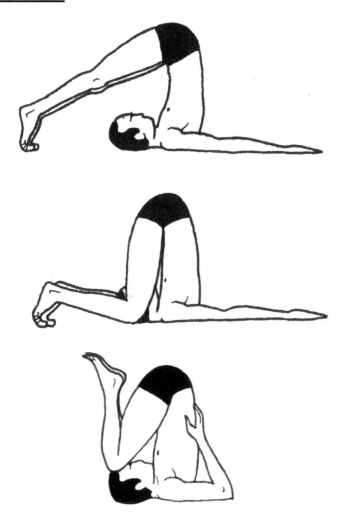

**DVI JANU SIRASA ASANA** Slowly come to *Dvi-Pada-Uttana-asana* on an in breath. Lift your buttocks and try to lift the legs behind the head to place the toes on the ground. Try to keep the spine straight and the back high without bending the legs. This is *Halasana*. Now bend your knees to place them against the ears, keeping the feet on the ground. Hold both the hands clasping the elbows over both legs. This is *Karana-Pira-asana*. Now place both the knees on your forehead keeping the feet straight over the head with the toes flexed back towards the head, soles to the sky. This is *dvi-janu-sirasa*-asana.

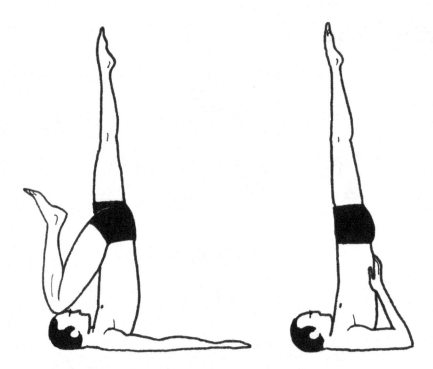

**EKA JANU SIRASA ASANA** From *Dvi-Janu-Sirasa-asana* slowly lift one leg straight up as high as possible, keeping the other leg in the previous position. This is *Eka-Janu-Sirasa-asana*. This is extremely good for the kidneys, pancreas, liver and spleen. It stimulates the blood flow in the pelvic region. Do the same asana on the other side.

**PROCESS** Slowly come to *Dvi-Pada-Uttana-asana* on an in breath. Lift your buttocks and try to lift the legs behind the head to place the toes on the ground. Try to keep the spine straight and the back high without bending the legs. This is *Halasana*. Now bend your knees to place them against the ears, keeping the feet on the ground. Hold both the hands from the elbows over both the legs tightly. This is *Karana-Pira-asana*. Now place both the knees on your forehead keeping the feet straight over the head with the toes flexed back toward the head, soles to the sky. This is *Dvi-Janu-Sirasa-asana*. Slowly straighten up both the legs and support the back with the elbows. Try to lift up the legs and back as high as possible. Your spine, buttocks and legs should be in the straight line. Chin should be locked into the collar bone. The whole of the body weight should be balanced on the shoulders. This is *Sarvangasana,* which is translated as all-limbs (in the air) posture. This should be included in regular practise as it is an asana that stimulates and activates all the limbs of the body.

**BENEFITS**

- This is very good for the pancreas, liver, spleen, stomach, thyroid and parathyroid glands. This is very good to control fat accumulation in the pelvic region.
- This asana can help prevent and cure epilepsy, constipation, headache, and ulcers of the intestines if practised carefully.
- It helps to stimulate the thyroid and thus helps maintain growth, metabolism and mental balance.
- Turning all the organs upside down creates an opportunity for them to readjust with gravity to where they should be.
- Young children who wish to increase their height should perform this asana.
- This asana benefits in asthma, bronchitis, and respiratory diseases.
- It is an important posture in *Kundalini* yoga and redirects lower energy to higher energy.

SPECIAL *Sarvangasana* is performed at the end of practise. It should be followed by *Matsyasana* and relaxation. For maximum benefits the whole series can be practised for five minutes or more. This asana has been recognised as very important in Hatha Yoga.

CAUTION Those who suffer from high blood pressure, heart diseases, or dizziness should perform this asana only under guidance.

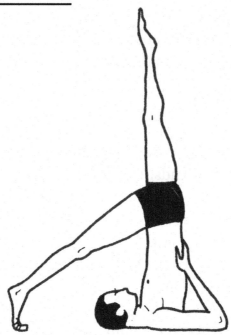

**EKA PADA SARVANGA ASANA** Perform *Sarvanga-asana* in the above vinyasa (series) and then place one leg on the ground as in *Halasana* and keep the other leg high in the *Sarvangasana* position. There should be no twist in your pelvic region while doing this asana. This is good to reduce fat accumulated in the pelvic region, hip area and thighs. This is very good for the liver and pancreas.

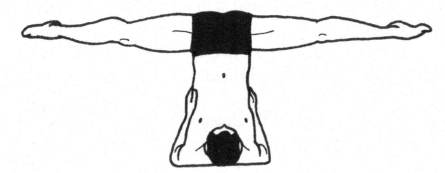

**SARVANGASANA PADAPRASARA** Perform the straight *Sarvanagasana*, support your back with both hands. Now slowly stretch down both legs to either side as far as you can. Try to keep the legs in a straight line.

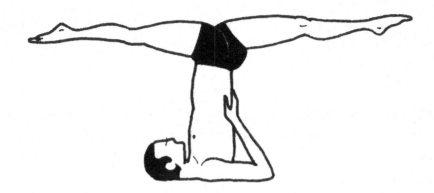

**SARVANGASANA PADAPRASAR PROVITTI** Perform the straight *Sarvanagasana* and support your back with both hands. Now slowly stretch down both legs; one leg in front and one behind the body. Let your legs reach a straight line in both directions with the buttocks as far as you can.

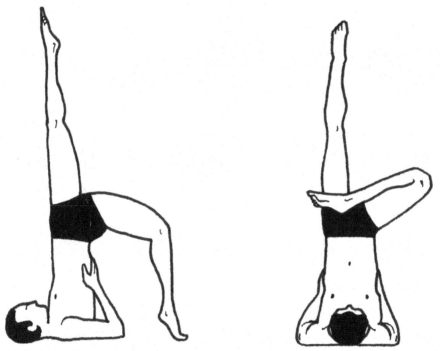

**SARVANGASANA EK PADA PRAVRITTI** Perform the straight *Sarvanagasana* and support your back with both hands firmly. Now slowly stretch down your right leg behind the body and try to place your foot on the ground; you can slightly bend your knee. Keep the left leg high and straight in the same *Sarvangasana* position. practise the same with the other leg.

**SARVANGASANA ARDHA PADMA** From *Sarvangasana* bring your right leg down to place the foot over the left thigh as in half-lotus, with keeping the left leg straight up. Hold it for few deep breaths and then repeat the same on the other side.

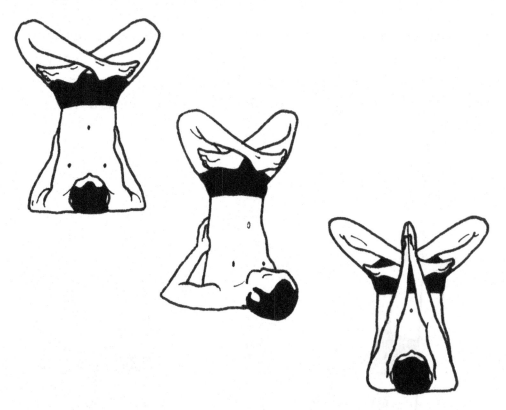

**SARVANGASANA PADMA** Place your right foot over your left thigh and then place your left foot over your right thigh as in *Padmasana*, keeping your knees pointing up. Repeat the same with left foot on right thigh.

**SARVANGASANA PADMA NIRALAMBA** From *Sarvangasana Padma*, if possible, stretch your hands in front of both knees and join them together in *Anjali Mudra*.

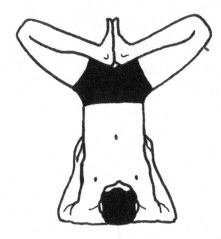

**SARVANGASANA BADDHA PADA** From *Sarvangasana,* open your knees out to
join both feet or soles together and bring them down close to groin
with keeping your knees opened out as in *Baddhakonasana.*

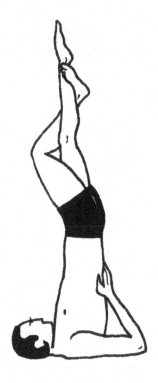

**SARVANGASANA GARUDA** In *Sarvangasana* bring your right leg in front
of your left and slightly bend it at the knee. Now twist your right
leg around left as far as you can as in *Garudasana* in standing.

If possible you can also practise *Niralamba* without the hands supporting the back, you can twist right hand around the left joining them in *Namaskar mudra*. Return back to *Sarvangasana* and repeat on the other side.

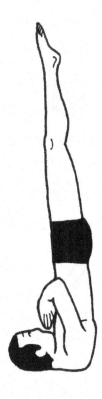

**SARVANGASANA NIRLAMBA** From *Sarvangasana* bring your hands in front and join them together in *Namaskar mudra* pointing to your chin and hold the mudra from 10 seconds to one minute.

**SARVANGASANA MAHABANDHA** All above variations can be practised with *Mahabandha, Moolabandha, Uddiyana Bandha,* and *Jalandhar bandha* together. These are specially beneficial for *Kundalini* awakening, redirecting lower energy to higher chakras and spiritual awakening. It recharges the body, mind and soul, refines *prana* and vital energy and establishes health, vitality, harmony and well being.

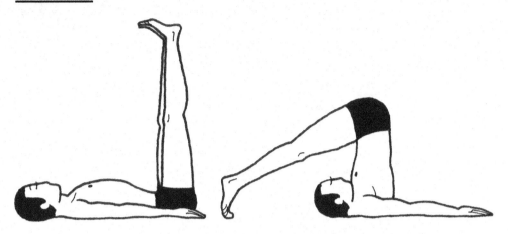

**PROCESS** Slowly come to *Dvi-Pada-Uttana-asana* on the in breath. Lift your buttocks and try to lift the legs behind and beyond the top of the head to place the toes on the ground. Try to keep the spine straight and back high without folding the legs. This is *Halasana*. Now you can use many different hand mudras and foot positions as variations of *Halasana*.

**HANDS VARIATION 1** Keep both hands straight on the ground behind the back with your palms to the ground.

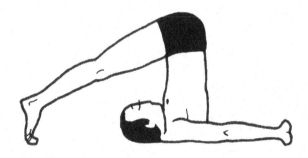

**HANDS VARIATION 2** Clasp the hands and stretch them straight on the ground behind the back with palms turned outward.

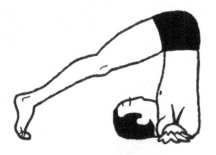 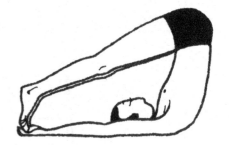

**HANDS VARIATION 3** Place the hands straight on the ground parallel to the shoulders with the palms to the ground.

**HANDS VARIATION 4** Keep both hands straight on the ground behind the head with palms the under the toes.

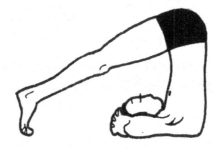

**HANDS VARIATION 5** Clasp the hands over the head.

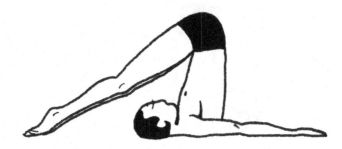

**LEGS VARIATION 6** Keep both hands in any of the above variations with both feet touching the ground with the soles facing upwards (i.e. toes are not tucked under).

**LEGS VARIATION 7** Keep both hands in any of the above variations with both feet touching the ground and heels are up and toes tucked under as in sitting in virasana like sitting in *Virasana* (ie toes are tucked under).

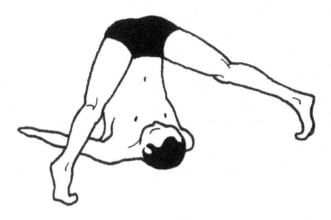

**LEGS VARIATION 8** Keep both hands in any of the above variations and stretch both the legs open (outwards) as much as possible. Your feet should be kept touching the ground and legs should be straight.

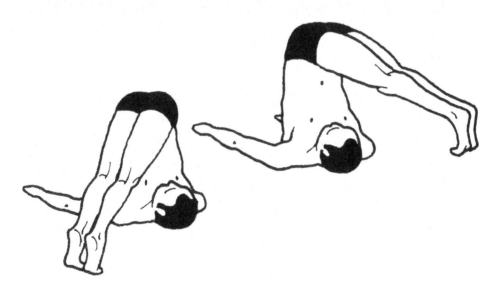

**LEGS VARIATION 9** Keep both the hands in any of the above variation and slowly rotate both the legs together first to the right side and then to the left side.

**BENEFITS**

- This asana stimulates, lengthens, and strengthens the back, shoulders, legs and all the associated muscles and ligaments.
- It removes constipation, increases digestive capacity, and balances thyroid hormones.
- This asana removes toxins accumulated in the spleen and kidneys.
- It can help to prevent and cure backache and neck-ache if practised cautiously.
- It regulates the blood circulation in all the parts of the abdomen, backbone, and the waist area.
- It eliminates fat on the belly and unnecessary fat over the buttocks and thighs.

SPECIAL In this posture the body takes the shape of a plough, or *Hal*asana. As per Tantra Yoga, this asana possesses a unique significance in restoring and refining sexual energy. This asana activates, strengthens, and rejuvenates all the sexual and reproductive organs. Because of this, it is very helpful in curing infertility.

CAUTION *Matsayasana* must be performed after this asana. Persons suffering from dizziness, heart problems, blood pressure problems, or spinal and shoulder injuries must perform this asana only under the guidance of a Yoga expert in a modified way.

DURATION Start with a few seconds, eventually this series of asanas should be performed for at least five minutes or more for better results.

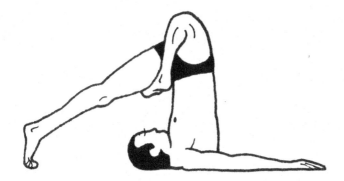

**HALASANA ARDHA PADAM** Come to *Halasana*, keeping your hands behind your back for support. Now bend your right leg and place your foot on your left thigh, keeping your knee over your head and the left leg straight. Repeat the same on the other side.

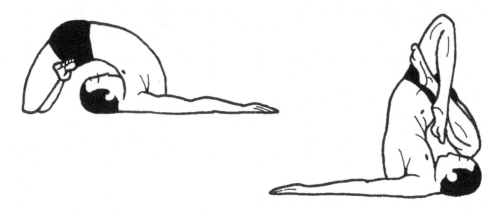

**HALASANA PADAM** As above, after placing the right foot against the left thigh, place the left foot on the right thigh. Keep both knees touching the ground. You can also practise *Padamasana* in a sitting position and then gradually come to *Halasana-padam*.

**HALASANA EKA JANU SIRSA PADAM** From the above *Halasana Padam,* twist from your hips and spine to place your right knee on your head with the left knee pointing upwards. Return back to centre and perform on the other side.

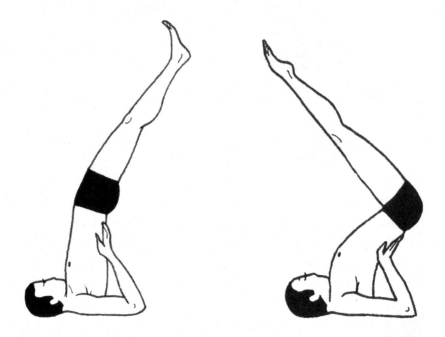

**PROCESS** Come to *Sarvangasana,* keeping your hands behind your back for support. Keeping your back and legs straight, slowly slightly bend from the torso to let your feet come over your head pointing to ceiling.

**BENEFITS** Along with all the benefits of *Sarvangasana* and *Halasana* this asana is particularly beneficial for the stomach and can cure and prevent ulcers and acidity problems if performed after drinking a glass of water.

**DURATION** Starting from few seconds, one should eventually hold this posture for three minutes or more.

## 57 KARAN PEEDASANA

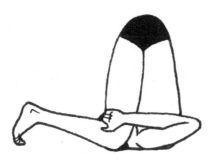

**PROCESS** Slowly come to *Dvi-Pada-Uttana-asana* on the in breath. Lift your buttocks and try to lift the legs behind the head to place the toes on the ground. Try to keep the spine straight and back high without bending the legs. This is *Halasana*. Bend your knees to place them against the ears, keeping the feet on the ground. Hold both the hands from the elbows over both the legs tightly. This is *Karana-Pira-asana*. Return to *Halasana* and then back to *Savasana*.

**BENEFITS**
- This is extremely good for the thyroid gland, throat, neck, all abdominal organs and ears.
- It increases the digestive strength and removes indigestion.
- It removes toxins accumulated in the kidneys, spleen, and pancreas.
- It helps to prevent backache and neck-ache. It regulates blood circulation in the whole body.
- It reduces or removes unnecessary fat accumulated on the belly, buttocks and the thighs.
- In young children this asana can help increase the height, cure ear problems, and prevent headache and migraine.

**CAUTION** *Matsyasana* must be performed after this asana. Those who suffer from chronic back, neck or shoulder problems should perform this asana under the supervision of a Yoga expert.

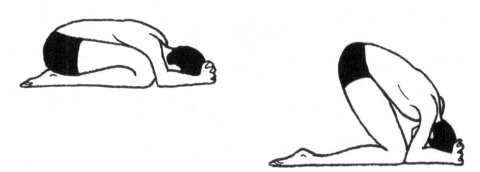

**PROCESS** Lock both your hands on the floor and open your elbows wide enough to make a triangle and place the top of your head on floor, in the middle.

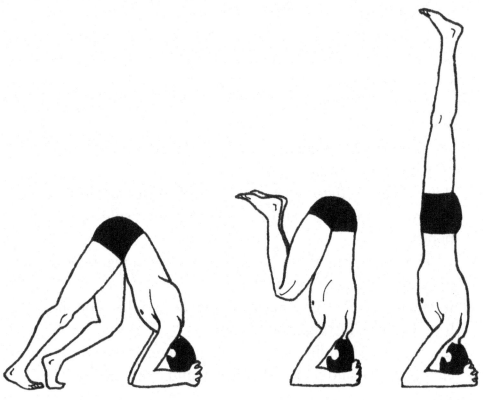

Slowly bend your knees and lift them over your head and gradually stretch them straight over as if you were standing straight from head to toe. Hold the posture and breathe deeply with *Sukha pranayama*.

**SPECIAL NOTE** *Shirshasana* is regarded as the king of asanas. There can not be a king without the subjects. Therefore, first the subjects i.e. perform well all the asanas before getting into *Shirshasana*. This will prepare the blood circulation, body fluids and prana to flow properly and maintain it against gravity. This asana reverses the general principle of gravity and all the parts of the body are affected by this single posture. This asana is difficult but one can achieve expertise by doing it regularly. If the balance is not maintained at the initial stage, one should take support of a wall or the assistance of a person.

## SHIRASHASANA VARIATIONS

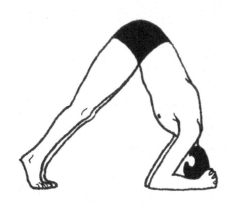 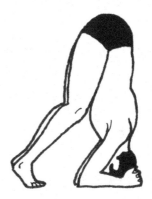

**SHIRASHASANA SAPURNA** For Yoga seekers who have neck, head and heart problems under control and like to benefit from *Shirashasana*, this is the variation to follow. As in *Shirashasana* once you place the top of your head on the floor, supported with hands and elbows in a triangle, slowly tuck your toes in on the floor and lift your knees up while bringing your legs straight. You can lift your knees up with the in breath and bring them down with the out breath or hold the posture from a few seconds to 30 seconds.

**SHIRASHASANA SAPURNA KRIYA** Once you have mastered the above one can start preparing for the next level towards *Shirashasana* with this kriya. Come to *Shirashasana Sapurna* and then walk your toes on the floor towards your head, allowing the knees and thighs to come close to the chest. Repeat it five to nine times.

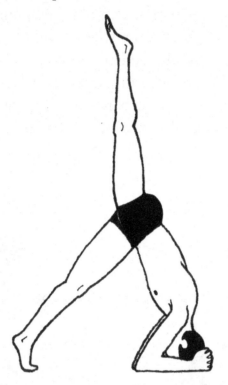

**SHIRASHASANA SAPURNA EKAPADA** Come to *Shirashashana Sapurna* and then lift your right leg straight up pointing up to the ceiling. Repeat the same with changed legs.

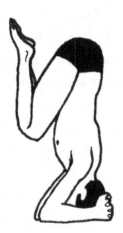

**ARDHA SHIRASHASANA** Continuing from *Shirashasana kriya* once your head and chest are close to the chest, using your pelvic and core muscles lift both your feet up and allow your knees to come on top of the head, with your feet pointing straight over.

**SHIRASHASANA PURNA** Once you can hold *Ardha-Sirashasana*, slowly try to lift and stretch both your legs straight over your head and hold the posture for a few breaths.

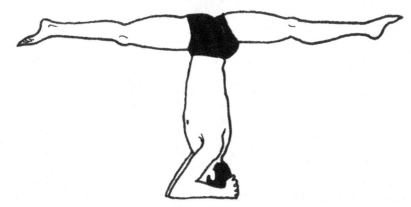

**SHIRSHASANA PADAPRASANA** Once you can hold to *Shirashasana Purna* slowly let your legs open out with the right leg to the front and left to the back, like coming to the splits. Repeat with switched legs.

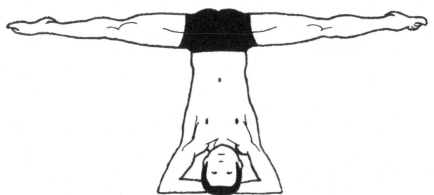

**SHIRSHASANA PADPRASARA PRAVRITTI** From *Shirashasana* now slowly open your legs out to the sides, as in side splits and hold the posture for few deep breaths.

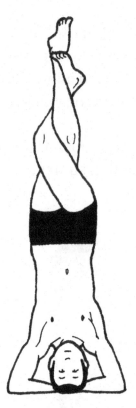

**SHIRSHASANA GARUDA** From shirashana bring your right leg in front of the left leg and wrap it around as in *Garudasana*. Repeat the same with switched legs.

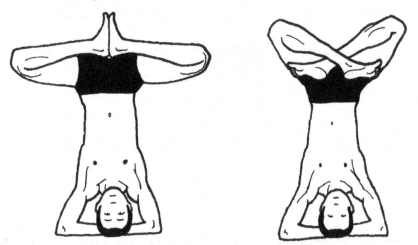

**SHIRSHASANA BADDHAPADA** From *Shirashasana* draw your feet down to your head joining both soles together and knees opened out wide.

**SHIRASHASHANA PADAM** Come to *Shirashasana* and slowly place your right foot on top of the left thigh and then place the left foot on top of right thigh, keeping the knees pointing over to the ceiling.

**BENEFITS**

- This asana regulates blood circulation in the pituitary gland and hypothalamus thus regulating complete body life mechanisms.
- Regular exercise of this asana prevents problems of the stomach, digestive system, back and conditions such as leprosy, jaundice and hernia.
- It stimulates the nervous system, refines the blood and naris and hence develops mental and emotional balance.
- It refines gross energy to pure prana or vitality and directs it from the lower to higher.
- It makes the body and energy attractive, light and radiant.
- It makes the body muscles strong and strengthens the head, neck, back, abdominal and pelvic muscles.

**CAUTION** Persons suffering from dizziness, heart problems, high blood pressure, brain or neck problems should perform this asana under strict guidance of a Yoga expert.

**DURATION** Begin it for a few seconds and practise the whole series for up to 10 minutes or more.

## 59 KAPALASANA

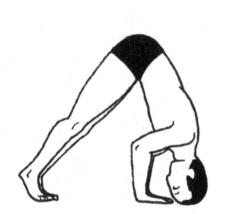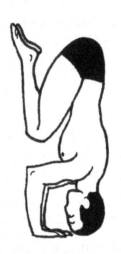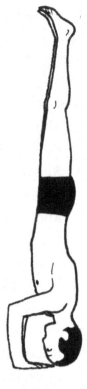

**PROCESS** Place the top of your head on a rug or soft Yoga mat while keeping both your hands on the floor to both sides with elbows up and pointing out. Slowly lift your legs over your head and stretch them straight over as in *Sirashasana*. Hold this posture for a few seconds to a minute.

**BENEFITS** Along with all the *Sirashasana* benefits it also establishes balance, harmony and homeostasis and builds will power and vitality. It helps opens the higher chakras and in-tunes with the higher consciousness.

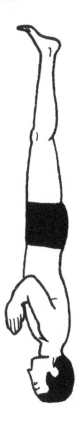

**PROCESS** Once you can hold *Kapalasana* easily, then slowly lift your hands over and join together in *Namaskar mudra* to your heart and hold from few seconds to a minute.

**BENEFITS** Along with all the *Sirashasana* benefits it also establishes balance, harmony and homeostasis and builds will power and vitality. It helps opening higher chakras and tuning into higher consciousness.

**CAUTION** *Kapalasana* and *Niralamba Sirashashana* should be practised only after mastering *Shirashana* properly.

## CHAPTER 10

# HAND OR ARM BALANCING POSTURES

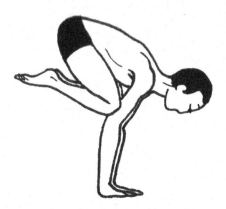

**PROCESS** Come to a squatting position and place both your palms on the floor in front of your knees. Keeping your elbows slightly bent, place both your knees on top of bent elbows on upper arms. Now slowly lift your feet up while balancing your whole body on both hands, supporting it with your knees against the elbows.

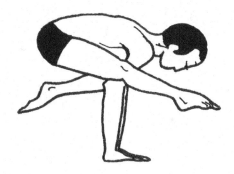

**BAKASANA SAPURNA** As above after placing your knees over your elbows try to lift one foot up and hold the posture. Repeat the same with the other leg.

**BAKASANA PURNA** From a squatting position open your knees and place your palms on the floor, locking your legs, thighs and arms against each other. Slowly come forward and try to lift your feet up and balance.

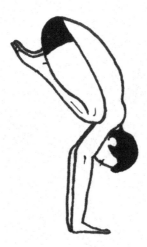

**BAKASANA SAMPURNA** If you can balance in *Bakasana* then gradually try to push your knees further up over your upper arms to your armpits and knees, feet pointing over your head.

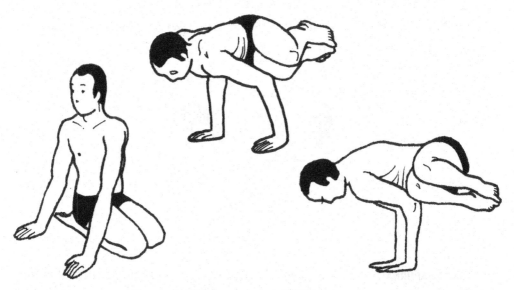

**PARSHVA BAKASANA** Come to *Vajrasana* or *Utkatasana* and place both your hands on the floor over the right side close to the thigh. Now slowly lift both your legs and hips up side-ways, using your right arm and elbow against your waist. Repeat the same to left side.

**SPECIAL** 'Baka' is a Sanskrit word, for 'heron'. This asana resembles a heron standing on both legs. Therefore, this asana is called '*Bakasana*'.

- This asana stimulates and strengthen abdominal and pelvic organs and muscles.
- It brings mental and emotional balance and increases memory.
- It opens the chest and heart and helps to build will power and confidence.
- It purifies the blood and stimulates the digestive system.
- It strengthens the arms and shoulders.

**CAUTION** Persons having dislocated joints or fractures should practise this asana under guidance in a modified approach.

**DURATION** Begin it for a few seconds and build up for up to three minutes.

## 62 BAKDHYANASANA

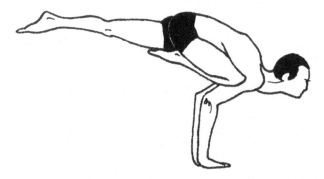

**PROCESS** Come to *Aradhpadmasana* in a squat with the right leg. Now as in *Bakasana* place your right knee on top of the left elbow or armpit and right leg over the right elbow. Slowly lift your feet and body up and stretch the left leg behind. Repeat the same with changed sides.

**NOTE** This is the meditative posture of a heron. The heron maintains the balance of the whole body on a single leg and remains in the

*Lakshabhed mudra* (a gesture for achieving the target), though looking inactive and calm to fishes, it catches them as they approach closer. 'Bakodhyanam' is counted among the five qualities required of a student to be successful.

**BENEFITS**
- It stimulates and strengthens the digestive and pelvic organs.
- It releases mental tension, fears, anxieties and increases memory.
- It strengthens the shoulders, arms, wrists and widens the chest.
- It purifies the naris and blood and charges the body, mind and soul with vitality.
- It strengthens the arms and the feet and develops balance.
- It helps building up core muscles, pelvic floor muscles and abdominal muscles.

**CAUTION** Practise this asana only after strengthening the wrists, elbows, arms and shoulders.

## 63 VRASHCHIKASANA

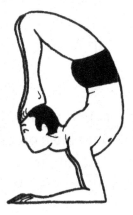

**PROCESS** Place both the palms and elbows on your Yoga mat firmly. Slowly lift both legs over your head, bend from the knees backwards and place your toes on top of the head.

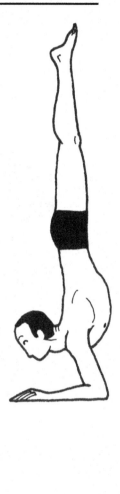

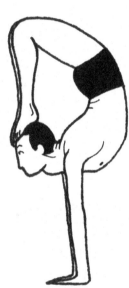

**VRASCHIKASANA SAPURNA** Placing both palms and elbows on the floor firmly with the in breath, lift up your legs over your head while keeping the legs straight and hold for few deep breaths. Return back with out breath.

**VRASCHIKASANA PURNA** Come to *Vrischikasana* while the toes touch on the top of head. Now slowly stretch your arms straight and hold your posture.

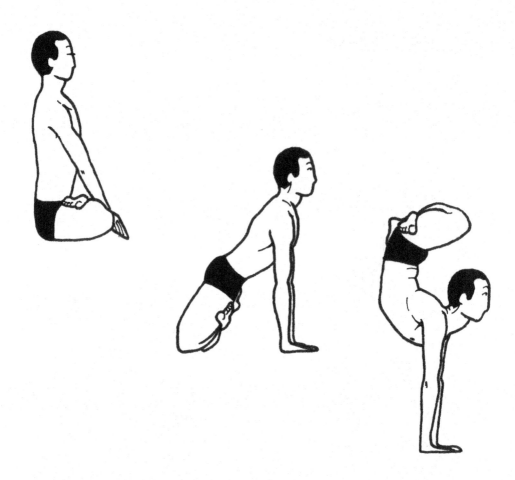

**VRASCHIKASANA PADMA** Sit up straight in *Padamasana* and place both your hands on floor in front and come on to the knees. Now slowly with the in breath lift your body up on your straight arms bringing your knees towards the head and hold to the posture. Return back with out breath.

**SPECIAL** *Vrashchikasana* means scorpion posture, i.e. drawing up asana resembling a scorpion.

**BENEFITS**
- This asana purifies the liver, kidneys, spleen and intestines.
- It increases digestive capacity and regulates the blood circulation.

- It makes the backbone strong and flexible. It removes stiffness, heaviness and lethargy from the whole body.
- It removes unnecessary fat.
- This asana prevents and cures mental lethargy and nervous weakness.

**CAUTION** Perform this asana only after attaining good mastery *Shalbhasana* series.

**DURATION** Begin for a few seconds and build the series for up to three minutes.

## 64 MAYURASANA

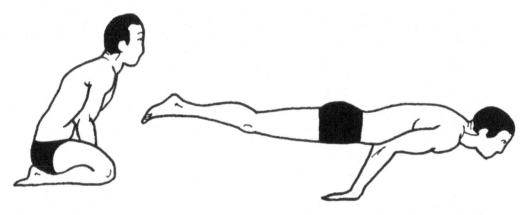

**PROCESS** Sit straight on the knees keeping hip space in between them. Bring together both the elbows and bend them. Place both palms on the ground with fingers pointing down towards the feet. Place your abdomen on both the elbows united under the navel. Slowly lift and stretch both your legs back while balancing your belly on your elbows, with the nose slightly above the ground. Gradually aim to bring your body straight in a straight line from head to feet.

## 65 MAYURIASANA

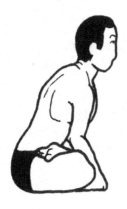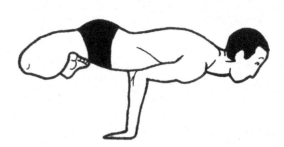

**PROCESS** Sit up straight in *Padmasana*. Place your hands firmly on the floor and abdomen on your elbows united together under the navel area. Slowly lift up in *Padmasana* and balance your body on your hands. The higher you bring up the legs, the more beneficial accordingly it would be with keeping your head above the ground too.

**BENEFITS**
- This asana strengthens the shoulders, elbows and the wrists.
- It stimulates and strengthens the liver, spleen, kidneys, stomach and intestines.
- It increases digestive capacity and cures lethargy, lack of energy and interest, indigestion and constipation.
- It refines and regulates blood circulation in the whole body.

**SPECIAL** According to the *Hatha Yoga Pradipika*, one who masters *Mayurasana* can digest lethal poison and any food.

**CAUTION** Do not perform any asana except the *Savasana* after *Mayurasana*. If you have had any surgeries in the abdomen or pelvic area perform this asana only under guidance.

**DURATION** Begin from a few seconds and build up to three minutes.

# ASANA PRACTICES AND SEQUENCES FROM LYING ON SIDE

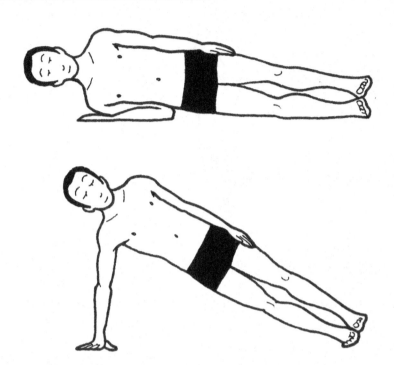

**PROCESS** Lay on your right side while keeping your left leg on the right leg and both legs straight. Place your right hand firmly on the floor and lift your body up with straight arms while balancing on the right hand and right foot.

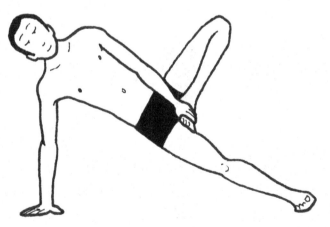

Now fold your left leg and hold your foot with the left hand.

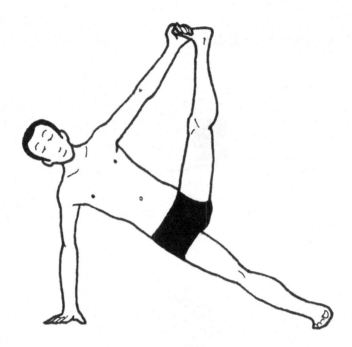

Stretch your leg straight over to the ceiling. Hold to your posture for few breaths and then return. Repeat the same on the left side.

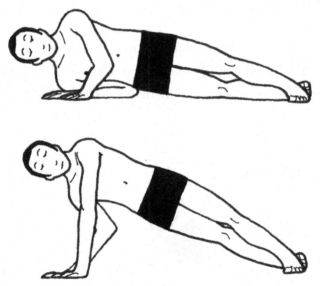

**VASHISHTHA TAPASYA ASANA SALAMBA** Lay on your right side and place your left foot on the floor in front of the right leg. Now place your left hand on floor in front of the chest and lift your body up from the floor while balancing on both hands and feet.

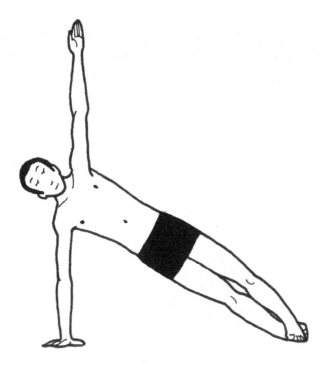

Now slowly lift your left hand up over your side pointing to ceiling. Repeat the same on the left side.

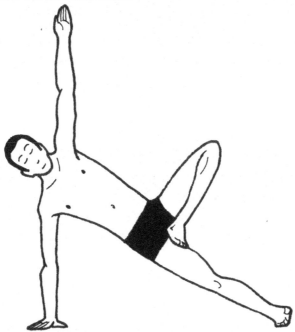

**VASHISHTHA TAPASYA ASANA SAPURN** From above once you feel comfortable, place your left leg on top of the right leg. Now balance on your right hand and foot with the left hand pointing over towards the ceiling. Repeat on both sides.

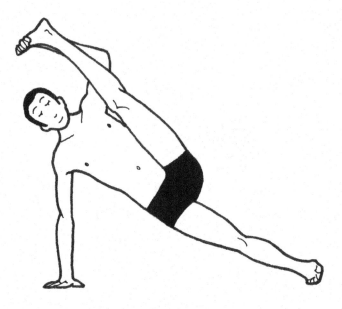

**VASHISHTHA TAPASYA ASANA SAMPURNA** Once you can hold *Vashishtha Tapasya asana* with your leg stretched over, gradually stretch and pull it further over your head. Repeat the same on both sides.

**BENEFITS**
- This series of postures balance right and left, loma-viloma, prana and apana and brings harmony or balance to the hormones and autonomic nervous system.
- It stimulates the nervous system and reactivates normal functioning of the body, mind and soul in harmony.
- It refines blood and naris and brings vitality and lightness.
- It strengthens shoulders, arms, wrists and waist areas.

**CAUTION** If you have injuries to the shoulders, arms, wrists or elbows practise this series under the guidance of a Yoga expert.

**DURATION** This series should be practised from a few seconds to five minutes for good benefits.

**SPECIAL** Sage Vashishtha used to meditate in this posture and realized truth and attained liberation and is hence known by his name.

## CHAPTER 12

# ASANA PRACTICES AND SEQUENCES FROM SHAVASANA (SUPINE)

# 67 CHAKRASANA

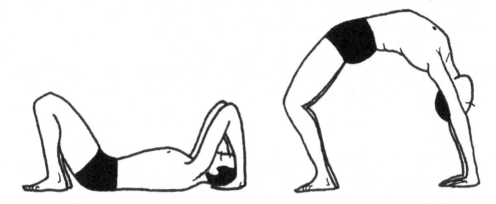

**PROCESS** Lie down on your back and fold the legs at the knees, bringing your feet close to the buttocks. Place your palms on the ground over your shoulders with the fingers pointing towards the shoulders and the elbows pointing straight up. Now slowly lift your shoulders and upper back up to place the top of your head on the floor. Press down firmly on your palms, fingers, and feet to lift whole body up, curving your whole body into a wheel and hence the posture is known as *Chakra-asana*.

**BENEFITS**

- This asana can help young children to increase height and strengthen muscles, joints and ligaments.
- Eliminates constipation and strengthens the abdominal and pelvic area and associated muscles.
- It refines energy and vitalizes the body and mind and makes the personality radiant. It beautifies the upper body of women and makes it strong.
- This asana provides a good stretch for the spine, shoulders, arms, neck and hips and all the associated muscles in these areas and strengthens them, and helps one to gain good control over their limbs and increases attentiveness and concentration.
- It prevents sugar problems, diabetes and heart problems.

- It helps prevent and cure mental and emotional instability and mood disorders.
- It prevents Parkinsons disease and nervous disorders.

**CAUTION** Any one suffering from tuberculosis of the bones, joint dislocation, high blood pressure, or heart troubles should not perform this asana or should practise in a modified and supported way under guidance.

**SPECIAL** *Paschimottasana* should be performed after *Chakrasana*. Young children should perform this asana from a standing position. The whole body assumes the shape of a circle in *Chakrasana*. This is a challenging asana and one need to be cautious. This requires a supple and strong body. The wheel is a symbol of movement, wealth, power and change. Vishnu's weapon 'Sudarshan chakra' is famous in Indian history as a symbol to conquer the demons and negative energy to support and enrich goodness and wealth. Likewise, the warriors' chariot wheel is also called 'Rath Chakra', a symbol of power and protection.

**DURATION** Begin it for a few seconds; eventually this asana series should be performed for five minutes for better results.

### CHAKRASANA VARIATIONS

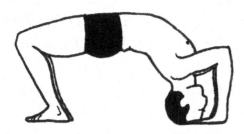

**CHAKRASANA SAPURNA** Lie down straight on your Yoga mat. Bend your legs at the knees bringing your heels close to the buttocks.

Bend your elbows over your head placing palms on floor close to shoulders with your fingers facing downwards. Now slowly lift your buttocks, back, chest and shoulders up, placing the top of the head on the floor. Pushing into the arms and legs in this position will help strengthen the body to prepare for full *Chakr*asana. Return back to *Shavasana*.

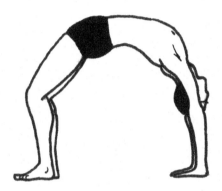

**CHAKRASANA PURNA** From the above position push further up on hands and feet to lift your head above the ground, curving the whole body. If possible walk your hands and feet further in so your arms are straight under the shoulders with the head hanging in between the arms. Lift up from the centre with your navel pointing up.

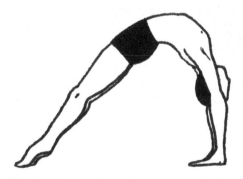

**CHAKRASANA PARIPURNA** From the above variation, walk your feet away from you, bringing legs straight and finally balancing on your toes and hands. Also, if you can try, to maintain your hands position under shoulders.

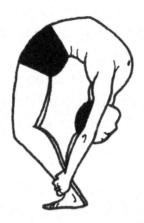 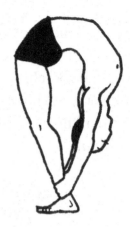

**CHAKRASANA SAMPURNA** From *Chakrasana Purna* stretch further up from the centre. Maintaining the balance gradually walk your hands towards feet and hold to your ankle joints.

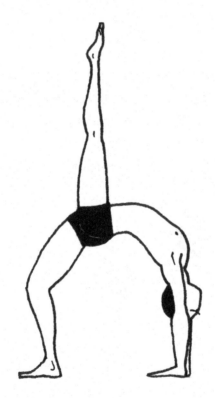

**CHAKRASANA EKA PADA** From *Chakrasana Purna*, if possible, lift one leg up with the foot pointing up. Return back to *Chakrasana* and repeat with the other leg.

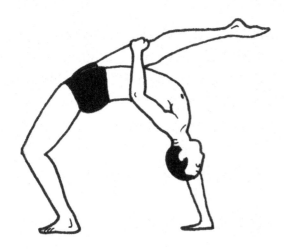

**CHAKRASANA EKA PADA EKA HASTA** As above, lift the right leg and left hand up with the aim to hold the leg over your chest. Return back to *Chakrasana* and repeat on the other side.

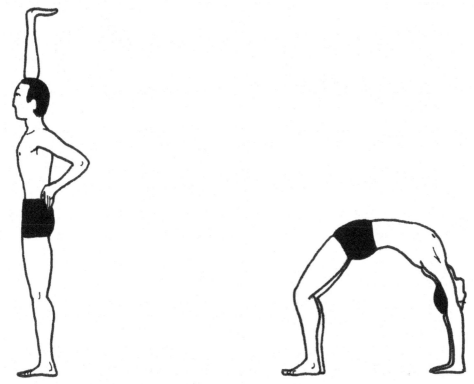

**CHAKRASANA FROM STANDING** Stand straight in *Samasthiti*. Place your left hand behind your back or buttock and lift your right hand straight over your head with palm flat and pointing up. Now slowly start bending back from the lower back and torso to place your hand down on floor overhead. Now also place your left hand on floor to come to *Chakrasana*. Once you build strength, flexibility and confidence you can bend back and perform with both hands overhead together. This posture is amazing beneficial for young children to develop strength, flexibility, control, and endurance. To complete your series practise all variations of *Paschimottanasana* followed by *Shavasana*.

## 68 MATSAYASANA

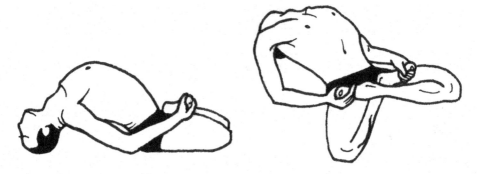

**PROCESS** Come to *Padmasana* and lie down flat on your back. Hold each foot with the same side hand, keeping the elbows on the ground close to your sides. Now gently lift up your shoulders and chest to place the top of your head on the floor with your chest wide open. Breathe deeply, engaging your mind around the heart area.

### BENEFITS
- This asana prevents and cures problems in the heart, lungs and neck.
- It opens mid-chest breathing and cures mental and emotional disorders. It also provides a good stretch for the abdominal muscles and stimulates them.
- This asana causes stretching of the neck and shoulder area as a contra-asana to the *Halasana* series, and *Sarvangasana* series.

- It brings vitality and lightness to body and mind.
- This develops the chest and the lungs, so it is very beneficial for asthma and cough.
- This asana prevents and cures disorders of the spleen.

**SPECIAL** This asana must be performed after *Sarvangasana* and *Halasana* series to balance the muscles and energy.

**CAUTION** Those who have serious neck injuries or problems should perform this asana only under guidance.

**MATSYASANA VARIATIONS**

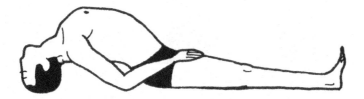

**MATSYASANA SAPURNA** Lie down flat on your back, keeping both legs straight and together. Now using both hands for support, place the top of your head on the floor, opening and lifting up the chest and shoulders. You can try to balance on the top of your head and buttocks here. Following are the hand variations.

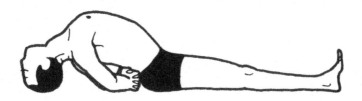

Place both hands on the thighs with elbows on the floor to either side. Interlock your hands under your mid and lower back area.

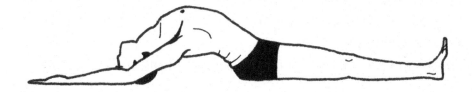

Stretch them on the floor straight over your head.

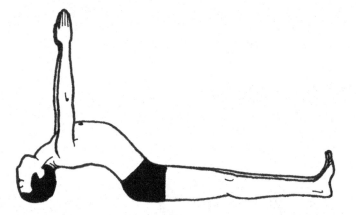

Stretch your arms straight over your heart and join together in *Agra mudra*.

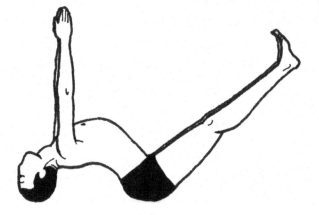

From position four, also lift your legs up feet pointing out around 45 to 60 degrees from the floor.

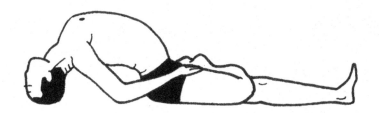

**MATSYASANA ARDHA PURNA** If you cannot do *Padamasana* then come to *Ardha-Padamasana* and practise *Matsyasana* with one of the hand variations.

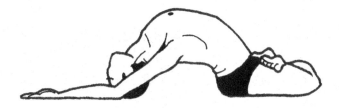

**MATSYASANA NIRALAMBA** Come to *Matsyasana* and then stretch your arms over your head on the floor. This asana forms the shape of a fish. The word 'Niralamb' means without support. Such an asana which is performed in this style without any support is called *'Niralamba Matsyasana'*.

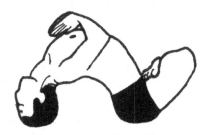

**MATSYASANA PARIPURNA** Come to *Matsyasana Niralamba* and join your hands together in *Namaskar mudra* to your heart. Now slowly lift up your knees and hips, maintaining the rest of the posture. You can use your hands for support to get to the position and then join them into *Namaskar mudra* or *Agra mudra*.

## 69 YOGANIDRASANA

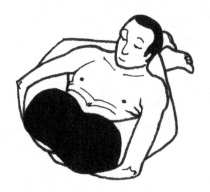

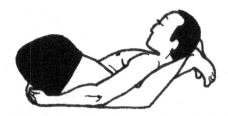

**PROCESS** Lie straight on your Yoga mat. Bring the left leg over and place your foot behind the neck and head, beneath the left shoulder. Likewise, bring the right leg over and place your foot behind the neck beneath the right shoulder. Let your head rest on your feet and neck on the cross point of the legs. Bring your hands behind your buttocks and interlock your fingers. You can hold this posture while holding the bandhas, for spiritual benefit and *Kundalini* awakening.

**BENEFITS**
- This asana is beneficial in awakening the *Kundalini*.
- This asana prevents and cures the problems related to the kidneys, spleen, intestine, stomach, genitals, and urinary track.
- It brings flexibility in the waist, neck, shoulders, legs and hips.

**CAUTION** This asana should be performed under guidance if you have dislocated joints or fractured and week bones.

**DURATION** Begin it from a few seconds, working towards three minutes.

## 70 SUPTA TRIKONASANA

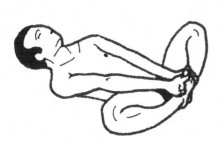 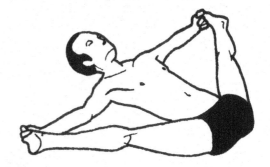

**PROCESS** Lie straight on your back. Bend both your knees to both sides and hold your big toes. Now slowly stretch both legs straight on the floor as in Padaprasa.

**NOTE** 'Supta' means to lie, and 'Trikona' means triangle. Here the body takes the shape of a triangle from the head to both feet and is known as *Supta-Trikonasana*. It's an important posture in Tantric traditions and the triangle base symbols the shakti, divine energy and the top edge represents shiva.

**BENEFITS**
- It stretches the lower parts of the body and opens the hips, stimulates and strengthens muscles and ligaments in the thighs, pelvis and hips.
- This asana can prepare women for easy delivery if practised before conception.
- Suppressed nerves between vertebrae resume a normal position and so removes associated pain.
- This asana is beneficial for the liver and the kidneys.

**CAUTION** This asana should be performed along with *Pada-Prasar* and *Hanumanasana*.

**DURATION** It should be performed from a few seconds to three minutes.

## 71 SUPTA TRIVIKRAMASANA

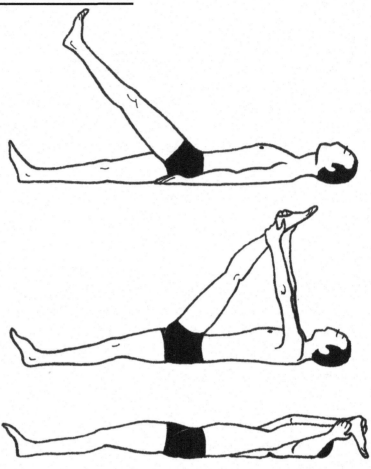

**PROCESS** Lie down straight on your back. With the in breath lift the left leg up and hold your leg or foot with both the hands. Now slowly bring your leg over your head and touch your toes to the floor, keeping both legs straight. Repeat the same with the right leg over the head and left straight down.

**BENEFITS**
- This asana stretches and stimulates hips, pelvic organs and muscles, lower back and ligaments through legs.

- It prepares for healthy pregnancy and helps in easy delivery if practised before conception.
- This asana is beneficial for strengthening the abdominal, pelvic and core area.
- It stimulates the nervous system and increases concentration, balance of mind and memory.
- This asana improves blood circulation in the feet, legs, thighs, and waist.

**CAUTION** Persons with back problems and weak joints should perform this asana under guidance.

**DURATION** Begin for a few seconds and try to master for three minutes.

## 72 NAVASANA

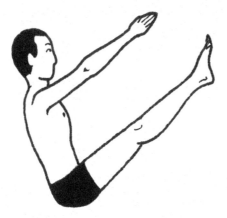

**PROCESS** Sit up straight from the *Savasana* and lift both your legs off the ground. Now shift both the hands parallel to the legs. The legs and hands should be on the same level. Try to keep the legs straight and balance the body on the tail bone. This is the simple *Navasana*. We can use many variations of the hand mudras in this; listed below. All have different therapeutic and spiritual aspects.

**NAVASANA MUDRA 1** Keep both the hands parallel to the legs with palms facing each other.

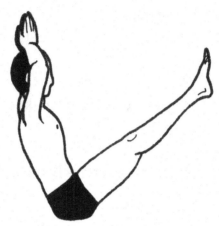

**NAVASANA MUDRA 2** Place both the hands over the head in *Anjali mudra*.

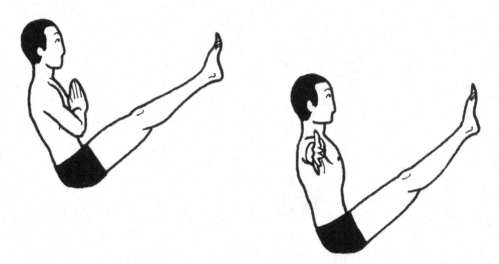

**NAVASANA MUDRA 3** Place both the hands in namaskar mudra in front of the chest.

**NAVASANA MUDRA 4** Turn both the hands parallel to the shoulders with palms facing front.

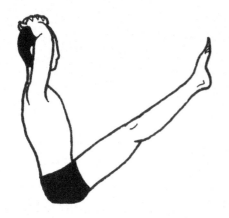 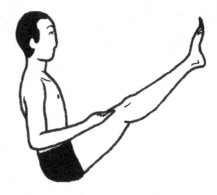

**NAVASANA MUDRA 5** Now clasp both the hands over the head.

**NAVASANA MUDRA 6** Finally place both the hands on the thighs.

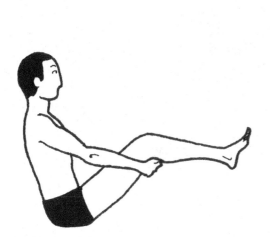 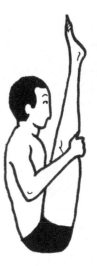

**NAVASANA SAPURNA** Sit straight with legs bent from the knees. Hold to your inner knees or thighs and slowly lean back on your tale bone to lift your feet above the ground with your in breath. Hold your position.

**NAVASANA SALAMBA** As above keep holding your inner knees or thighs and stretch your legs further up straight and hold your supported *Navasana*.

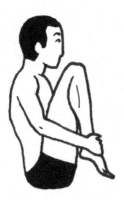

**NAVA ASANA SALAMBA PURNA** Sit up straight from *Savasana* and lift both of your legs from the ground, keeping the hands parallel to the legs. Now fold your legs and catch the ankles and stretch again into the *Navasana*. Balance your body on the tail bone and try to keep the knees straight.

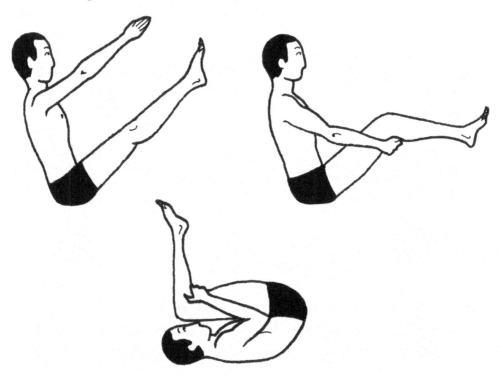

**NAVA ASANA KRIYA** Sit up straight from *Savasana* and lift both of your legs from the ground keeping the hands parallel to the legs. Now fold your legs and catch the knees from the inner side and roll on your back. Try to place your knees on the head, as in *Pavana-Mukta-asana* but keeping the feet high. Roll back and stretch again to *Navasana* (there is a similar kriya called *Gardhabha kriya* which uses sound with it).

**BENEFITS**
- This asana helps build up core strength and stimulates and strengthens abdominal and pelvic muscles.
- It stimulates and balances digestive secretions and helps prevent and cure abdominal problems.
- It stimulates and strengthens the pelvic organs, kidneys, adrenal glands and helps maintain their health.
- It refines gross energy to higher energies and brings vitality.
- *Navasana* is also an important posture in awakening the lower chakras or *Kundalini*.

# 73 SARVA ASANA

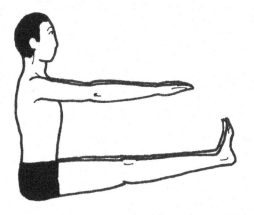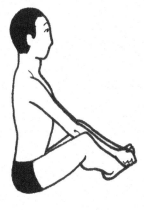

**PROCESS** Sit up straight from the *Savasana* and lift both of your legs from the ground whilst keeping the hands parallel to the legs. Now fold your legs and catch the feet from the inner side and stretch the legs apart. Try to keep the spine straight and the whole body balanced on the tale bone.

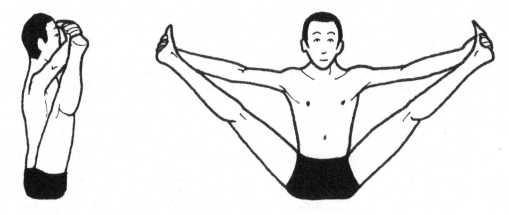

Balance your body on the tale bone and try to keep the knees straight and feet to shoulder or head height.

### BENEFITS
- This asana helps open the hips and stimulates the lower back, pelvic and abdominal area.
- This asana helps with preventing and curing reproductive organs and is recommended before and during pregnancy to prepare for easy delivery.
- It helps open the shoulders and widens the chest for deep breathing.
- It helps establishing balance, stability and concentration.

DURATION From 30 seconds to three minutes for good results.

CAUTION People suffering with serious back, hips or shoulder issues should practise it under guidance.

## 74 SETUBANDHASANA

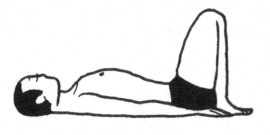

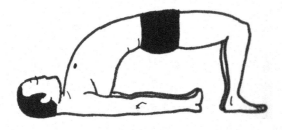

**PROCESS** Lie down straight on your back. Lift up your body from the middle, balancing on the heels and shoulders, coming to a bridge shape. You can keep your palms on the floor or interlock both hands under you back and stretch them inside out.

### SETUBANDHASANA VARIATIONS

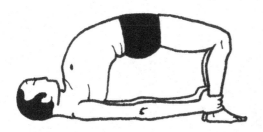

**SETUBANDHASANA SAPURNA** From a straight lying position bend your legs from the knees, drawing your heels to the buttocks. Hold your ankle joints or let your fingers point to your feet. Now slowly lift up your buttocks and back as far as you can. You can hold the posture for few breaths or lift up with the in breath and return with the out breath for few rounds. If you can, now interlock both your hands under your back and repeat the posture again.

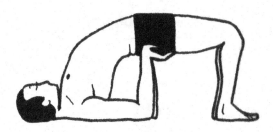

**SETUBANDHASANA SALAMBA** Come to *Setubandhasana Sapurna* and then place both your hands under your buttocks or sides, drawing your elbows to the floor beneath your hands to lift your body further up in *Setubandhasana*.

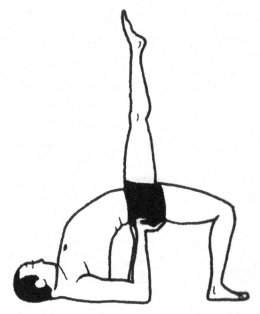

**SETUBANDHASANA SALAMBA EKAPADA** Come to *Setubandhasana Salamba* and then slowly with the in breath lift your right leg up straight pointing to the ceiling. Hold to your posture. Repeat the same with the left leg stretched over.

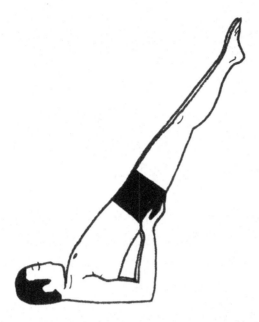

**SETUBANDHASANA SALAMBA DVIDAPA** Come to *Setubandhasana Salamba* and slowly draw your knees over and then stretch your legs behind in line with your chest, abdomen and pelvis.

**BENEFITS**

- This asana strengthens spine, hips, pelvis and abdominal organs.
- This asana is beneficial for the areas of the head, neck, shoulders and the waist.
- It prevents and cures arthritis and rheumatism.
- It regulates the blood circulation and stimulates spinal neurons and the nervous system.
- It is beneficial in backache and sciatica.

**CAUTION** Those who are overweight should be cautious with this asana, because there is a possibility of sprain or over straining in the wrists and elbows.

**DURATION** This asana series should be performed for three to five minutes.

## 75 PAVAN MUKTASANA

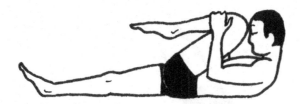

**EKA PADA PAVANA MUKTA ASANA** Lie flat on your back. Now bend the left leg slowly at the knee, bringing it over the chest, and hold it tightly with both hands. Now lift the head up slowly and touch the chin to the knee. Practise the same with the left leg.

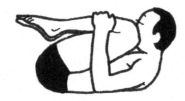

**DVI PADA PAVANA MUKTA ASANA** Lift and bend both legs together, bringing the knees over the chest and hold them tightly with both hands. Now with the out breath bring your chin to rest between the knees.

**BENEFITS**
- This benefits those who are suffering from constipation, indigestion, intestinal gas, and belching.
- This is beneficial for the digestive system.
- It prevents lung and heart diseases.
- It removes toxins accumulated in the ankles, knees, spine and thighs, and makes them supple.
- This asana removes toxins accumulated in the liver, spleen, stomach, and the kidneys etc.
- It can help to reduce flatulence and cure piles.

**SPECIAL** *Pavan Muktasana* relieves fat and gas accumulated in the abdominal area. If you are suffering with constipation it can be very beneficial if performed after drinking two glasses of water.

**DURATION** Repeat this asana twice or more, resting in between if needed.

## 76 SHAVASANA

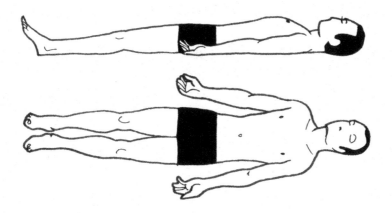

**PROCESS:** *Shava* means a corpse. In this asana, the body position resembles death. Every part of the body becomes still. In this asana, lie flat on the back. There should be a little gap in between the heels and the feet can fall gently outwards to either side. The palms should remain open, upwards, and close to the body. The head and the torso should be straight and the eyes gently closed. Now you can use auto-suggestion or a visualisation technique to relax every part of your body, one at a time, beginning at the toes.

**BENEFITS** This is a very important asana and practise for physical, mental, emotional and spiritual therapeutic purposes.

**CAUTION** Ideally one should never leave out this practice as it is here is that your body will benefit most to complete your hatha yoga practice. Try to maintain an even pattern of respiration, as this is necessary in *Shavasana*.

**SPECIAL** This asana reabsorbs the energy consumed in performing other asanas. Stretching or pain caused by asanas is removed. In the beginning, this asana should be performed after every other asana so that fatigue is avoided. When you are strong and full of energy, perform this asana after all the other asanas. This asana looks simple but it is considered an important one.

**DURATION** This asana should be performed for five minutes or more. The duration may be just one minute, if it is performed in between other asanas.

## CHAPTER 13

# CLASSICAL SITTING POSTURES FOR MEDITATION

## 77 PADMASANA

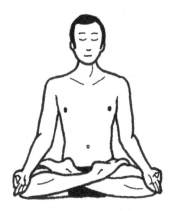

**PROCESS** Sit straight on your mat with your legs stretched forwards. Now gently bend your left leg at the knee and place your left foot on the right thigh. Now slowly bend your right leg and bring your right foot to the left thigh. Try to keep yours knees close to the floor. Place both your hands on your knees in *Jnana mudra*, keeping the back straight. Release from the posture and practise with the right leg first.

**BENEFITS**

- In this asana the spinal cord remains straight hence it is one of the important meditative postures in yoga.
- It re-aligns the hips, knees, thighs, legs and ankle joints as they should be on the floor.
- It cures skin diseases, cleanses the blood, *prana* and vital energies.
- It brings the sciatic nerve back to normal functioning.

**SPECIAL** This asana is suitable for pranayama and meditation. This asana eliminates restlessness of the mind and increases concentration. This asana takes the shape of a lotus; therefore, it is called *Padamasana*. As per Puranas, the Yogi becomes completely free from worldly bondages by performing pranayama in *Padmasana*. It is mentioned in the 'Goraksha Samhita' that

"Aasanan, dwividhan, proktan, padaman, *Vajrasana*", meaning thereby that only the two asanas are of prime importance: *Padmasana* and *Vajrasana*.

**CAUTION** If you not are used to sitting on the floor, this can be one of the most difficult postures to practise and you need to be patient and careful as its easy to dislocate ankle joints, or sprain muscles. In the beginning you can practise *Ardha-Padmasana*.

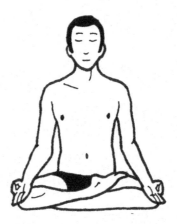

**ARDHA PADMASANA** Sit straight on your mat with your legs stretched forward. Bend your right leg and bring your foot under the left side. Now gently place your left foot on your right thigh, keeping the knee down on the floor. Repeat the same with your right foot on your left thigh.

**DURATION** This asana is for pranayama and meditation, hence one eventually needs to master it for a minimum of 48 minutes up to three hours or more.

## 78 BADDHPADMASANA

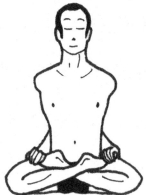

**PROCESS** Sit straight in *Padmasana*. Bring the right hand from behind to reach around to hold to your right foot or toes. Now reach your left hand around your back to hold to your left foot or toes. Breath slowly and deeply, equally into the lower, mid and upper lobes of your lungs while holding *Mulabandha*.

**SPECIAL** This asana is like an unfolded or unopened lotus and hence is known as *Baddha-Padmasana*. It refines and reserves or introverts the *prana* or vital energy and transcends it from the lower to higher chakras and is a very important posture in *Kundalini* awakening.

**BENEFITS**
- The spinal cord remains straight so it is ready for channeling *Kundalini* energy.
- It stimulates and strengthens the lungs and heart energy and balances them.
- It cleanses the blood and fluid systems by activating the kidneys, lungs, spleen and heart and thus prevents and cures skin diseases, blood disorders, respiratory disorders, and weakness and lethargy.
- It prevents and cures back, stomach and shoulder problems.
- It is a good stretch for the arms, shoulders, hips, knees and ankle joints and associated muscles.

**CAUTION** If you have serious injuries or fractures of the bones in the hands, shoulders, knees, or feet, you should perform this asana only under guidance in a modified way.

**DURATION** Begin for half a minute and gradually try to increase up to a few hours, holding bandhas with the order of breath.

## 79 VAJRASANA

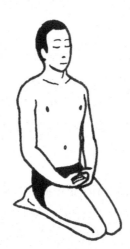 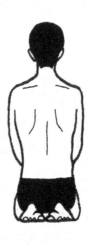

Sit down and fold your legs backward under your buttocks. Keep the heels and the toes together with flat feet. Slowly sit up, placing your buttocks on the heels. Place both your hands on your lap with the right hand on top, and thumbs touching each other. A Yoga seeker planning to learn pranayama especially needs to master this posture.

**BENEFITS**
- It stimulates and balances the digestive system.
- Naturally this enables one to sit straight with a straight spine as well as leaving the abdominal and diaphragmatic muscles free to allow the breath to flow freely in each section of the lungs.
- This asana enables diaphragmatic breathing to be properly active which also gives a good movement and massage to the stomach, gall-bladder, liver and intestines. This helps prevent

abdominal problems.
- This asana prevents diabetes.
- Increases concentration and memory.

**CAUTION** Those who have fractured or dislocated their ankle, knee, or hips should perform this asana only under guidance.

**SPECIAL** This is the only asana which can be performed after meals. This asana gives tremendous strength to the body. Vajra means thunderbolt. The heels pressing against the buttocks stimulates *Vajra-nari*, responsible for electromagnetic energy.

**DURATION** Start for a few seconds. Eventually, for full benefits this asana should be performed for five minutes or more.

### VAJRASANA VARIATIONS

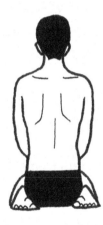 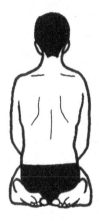

**VAJRASANA SAPURNA** From a kneeling position open your feet and gently sit down, placing your buttocks down on the floor with both feet tucked close to each side. Hold both hands together on your lap in *Dhyana mudra* with your spine straight and chin up .

**VAJRASANA PURNA** From a kneeling position, touch the big toes together and flatten your feet to each side making a v-shape. Now gently sit in the middle of the v-shaped feet. Hold hands in *Dhyana mudra*.

## 80 GORAKSHASANA

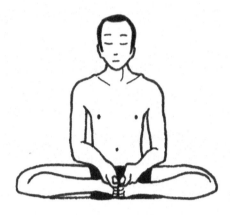 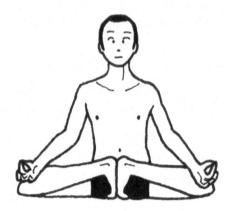

**PROCESS** Sit up straight in *Baddhakonasana*. Slowly come forward on your knees and let your heels come together over your genitals. Finally, your knees, both buttocks and toes are on the floor with your joined soles hiding your genitals. Place both hands on the knees in *Jnana mudra*. Try to hold your breath for few seconds up to three minutes and gaze on the tip of your nose while holding *Moolabandha* for *Kundalini* awakening.

**BENEFITS**
- This asana refines gross energies to subtle and vital energies and brings health, vitality and peace.
- It prevents and cures all sorts of sexual disorders in men and women and it is even mentioned in scriptures that it can cure infertility.
- It cures all the diseases related to kidneys and bladder.
- It cleanses naris, stimulates the lower chakras and leads to *Kundalini* awakening.

**CAUTION** This asana should be performed under guidance if you have ankle or knee joint problems.

**DURATION** Begin for a few seconds and build up to three minutes.

## 81 KANDPEEDASANA

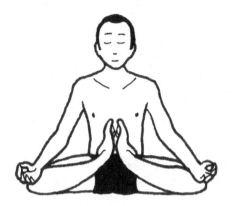

**PROCESS** Sit up straight with soles joined together. Now slowly lift your feet up together over your navel with turning your soles outwards. Place your hands on your knees in *Jnana mudra*, breath out fully and hold *Moolhabandha* as long as you can hold your breath out.

**SPECIAL** When *Kandpeedasana* is mastered, the *Kundalini* awakens naturally and travels up to the Brahmrandra (top of the head). This is the goal of our Yoga practise.

**BENEFITS**
- This asana helps improve flexibility of the ankles, knees and hips and brings them to the natural form we are born with.
- It eliminates toxins from thighs, legs, knees, pelvis and abdominal area.
- This asana purifies gross energies and refines them to higher energies.
- It stimulates abdominal and pelvic organs and cures all the associated problems.
- This asana is also a preventive and curative posture for reproductive organs in men and women.

## 82 SUKHASANA

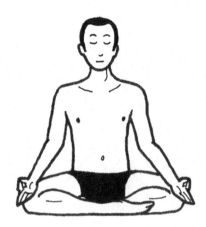

**PROCESS** Sit straight with legs bent in front. Now cross your legs with both feet on the floor and let the knees come down to the floor. Place your hands on your knees in *Jnana mudra* or your lap in *Dhyana mudra*.

**SPECIAL** Term shukha means easy or pleasant. This is a comfortable seated posture and in generally used for building long sitting postures like *Padmasana, Vajrasana,* or *Siddhasana* as a transitional posture to relax ankle joints.

**BENEFITS**
- Helps realigning hips, knees and ankle joints on the floor.
- It is good for relaxing and stilling our body, mind and senses.

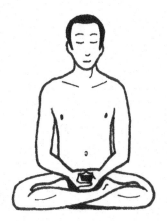

**PROCESS** Sit straight with legs stretched in front. Bend both your knees to come to a cross leg position, keeping your knees up. Now tuck both your feet inside your knees in between the calf and thigh muscles, to hide your toes. Place both the knees down on the floor and hands on your lap, with the right hand on top and thumbs touching each other in *Dhyana mudra*.

**BENEFITS**
- This is one of the meditative postures and helps sadhaka to be stable, firm and comfortable and to sit straight.
- This asana helps align the knees, hips, and ankle joints on the floor as they should be.
- It helps increase concentration and memory.

**DURATION** This asana should be mastered from three to 48 minutes or more for desired benefits.

## 84 SIDDHASANA

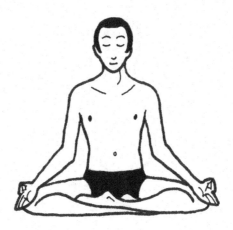

Process- Sit straight with legs stretched in front. Fold your right leg and place your heel against the groin under the genitals. Now fold your leg to place your foot on top of the right foot over the genitals. Place both hands on your knees in *Jnana mudra* or on your lap in *Shakti mudra*.

### BENEFITS

- This is another meditative posture and helps the sadhaka to awaken *Kundalini* or vital energy and transforms lower energy to higher energy.
- It also helps the holding of *Moolabandha* for longer periods as it locks the points in the posture itself and hence transcends the mind from the lower to higher chakras or energy channels.
- It helps improve vitality, health, well being and concentration if practised regularly and removes lethargy, stress, mental imbalances, agitation, irritation, etc.

DURATION This asana should be mastered from three minutes to 48 minutes.

**AHAMKARA** Ego.

**AHIMSA** Non violence, harmlessness (one of the yamas).

**AKASHA** Space; ether,

**ANANDA.** Bliss, joy.

**APARIGRAHA** Nongreed (one of the yamas).

**ARJUNA** One of the five Pandava back brothers; he whom Lord Krishna Addressed the Bhagavad Gita.

**ASANAS.** Yoga postures, 3rd limb of ashtanga yoga.

**ASHRAM** Retreat or secluded place, usually where the principles of yoga and meditation are taught and practiced.

**ASHTANGA** Eight limbs Ashtanga yoga. Eightfold path of yoga, Raj Yoga of Patanjali with eight limbs-yamas, Niyamas, etc.

**ASMITA** Ego, individuality, I-am-ness.

**ASTEYA** Nonstealing (one of the yamas).

**ATMA** Soul, individual spirit.

**BHAKTA** Devotee.

**BHAKTI** Devotion.

**BHAKTI YOGA** The path of devotion.

**BRAHMACHARYA** Purity, chastity (one of the yamas).

**BRAHMAN** The absolute. Divinity itself, God as creator.

**BUDDHI** The intellect.

**CHAKRAS** Centers of radiating life force or energy that are located between the base of the spinal column and the crown of the head. Sanskrit for "wheels". There are seven chakras that store and release life force (prana).

**CHETANA** Consciousness, awareness.

**CHIT** Eternal consciousness.

**CHIT-SHAKTI** Mental force governing the subtle dimensions.

**CHITTA** Individual consciousness including the subconscious and unconscious levels of mind, memory, thinking, attention, etc.

**CHITTA-VRITTI** Mental modifications.

**DEVATA** Deity

**DEVI** Female deity, goddess.

**DHARANA** From the word dhri

meaning "to hold firm," this is concentration or holding the mind to one thought.

**DHARMA** Self-discipline, the life of responsibility and right action.

**DHYANA** Meditation or contemplation. The process of quieting the mind.

**DIVYA** Divine

**DOSHAS** Impurities or deformities in body, mind or emotions.

**DRASHTA** Seer, observer, awareness.

**DRISHTI** Vision.

**GAYATRI MANTRA** Vedic mantra of 24 matras or syllables invoking the pure eternal energy.

**GHERANDA SAMHITA** Traditional yogic text of Rishi Gheranda. Guru. Spiritual teacher.

**HATHA YOGA** It is the yoga of physical well-being, designed to balance body, mind, and spirit.

**INDRIYAS** Sense organs.

**ISHVAR-PRANIDHANA** Surrender to God (one of the niyamas).

**IYENGAR YOGA** This yoga style focuses on the body and how it works. It is noted for attention to detail, precise alignment of postures, and the use of props.

**JIVA** Individual life

**JIVAN** Life.

**JNANA** Knowledge or wisdom.

**JNANA YOGA** The path of knowledge or wisdom.

**KAIVALYA** State of consciousness beyond quality.

**KALA** Time.

**KAMA** Desires.

**KARMA** Action, law of cause and effect which shapes the destiny of each individual.

**KARMA YOGA** The path of action.

**KARMENDRIYAS** Five physical organs of action- feet, hands, speech, excretory and reproductive organs.

**KIRTAN** Singing holy songs.

**KOSHAS** Body, sheaths.

**KRIYA** Motion, movement.

**KUNDALINI** A cosmic energy in the body that is often compared to a snake lying coiled at the base of the spine, waiting to be awakened. Kundalini is derived from kundala, which means a "ring" or "coil."

**KUNDALINI YOGA** Chanting and breathing are emphasized over postures in this ancient practice designed to awaken and control the release of kundalini energy.

**LAYA** To dissolve.

**LAYA YOGA** Yoga of conscious dissolution of individuality.

**LOKAS** Seven planes of consciousness.

**LORD KRISHNA** Because of his great Godly power, Lord Krishna is another of the most commonly worshipped deities in the Hindu faith. He is considered to be the eighth avatar of Lord Vishnu. Shree Krishna delivered Bhagvad Gita on battlefield of Mahabharata to Arjun.

**MALA** Garland.

**MANAS** Mind.

**MANDALA** A circular geometric design that represents the cosmos and the spirit's journey. It is a tool in the pilgrimage to enlightenment.

**MANTRA** Sacred chant words.

**MAUNA** Silence.

**MAYA** Illusion.

**MITAHARA** Balanced diet.

**MOKSHA** Liberation.

**MUDRAS** Hand gestures that direct or control the life current through the body.

**MUKTI** Liberation.

**NADA** Pranic or psychic sound.

**NADI** Channels of pranic/psychic energy flow.

**NAMASTE** This Hindu salutation says "the divine in me honors the divine in you." The expression is used on meeting or parting and usually is accompanied by the gesture of holding the palms together in front of the bosom.

**NIDRA** Sleep.

**NIRBIJA SAMADHI** Final state of smadhi where there is absorption without seed; total dissolution.

**NIRVICHAR SAMADHI** Transitional state of Samadhi; absorption without reflection.

**NIRVIKALPA SAMADHI** Transitional state of Samadhi involving purification of memory, which gives rising to Jnana or true knowledge.

**NIYAMAS** In the Yoga Sutras, Patanjali defined five niyamas or observances relating to inner discipline and responsibility. They are purity, contentment, self-discipline, study of the sacred text, and living with the awareness of God.

**OM OR AUM** Mantric word chanted in meditation. Paramahansa Yogananda called it the "vibration of the Cosmic Motor." This one word is interpreted as having three sounds representing creation, preservation, and destruction.

**PANCHA-KLESHA** Five afflictions – ignorance, ego, attraction, aversion and fear of death.

**PATANJALI** Ancient Rishi who codified the ashtanga yoga known as Yoga-Sutra.

**PRAKRITI** Nature.

**PRANA** Life energy, life force, or life current vital energy; inherent vital force pervading every dimension of matter.

**PRANAVA** Mantra AUM; primal sound vibration.

**PRANAVA DHYANA** Meditation on the mantra AUM.

**PRANAYAMA** Method of controlling prana or life force through the regulation of breathing.

**PRATYAHARA** Withdrawing the senses in order to still the mind as in meditation.

**PURUSHA** Individual Soul or spirit.

**RAJA YOGA** The path of physical and mental control.

**RISHI** Realized sage, one who meditate on Self.

**SABEEJA SAMADHI** Absorption with seed where the form of awareness remains.

**SADHAKA** Spiritual aspirant.

**SADHANA** Spiritual practice.

**SAHAJA.** Spontaneous, easy.

**SANTOSHA** Contentment (one of the niyamas).

**SATYA** Truthfulness and honesty (one of the yamas).

**SAMADHI** State of absolute bliss, superconsciousness (8th limb of ashtanga yoga).

**SHAUCHA** Purity, inner and outer cleanliness (one of the niyamas).

**SHAT-DARSHANAS** Six Ancient Indian philosophies about truth or reality.

**SWADHYAYA** Self-study. The process of inquiring into your own nature, the nature of your beliefs, and the nature of the world's spiritual journey (one of the niyamas).

**SWAMI** Title of respect for a spiritual master.

**TAMAS** One of the three gunas; state of inertia or ignorance

**TANTRA YOGA** This yoga uses visualization, chanting, asana, and strong breathing practices to awaken highly charged kundalini energy in the body.

**TAPAS** Self-discipline or austerity (one of the niyamas).

**UPANISHADS** Vedantic texts conveyed by ancient sages and seers containing their experiences and teachings on the ultimate reality

**VAIRAGYA** Non-attachment.

**VAISHESHIKA** A treatise on the subtle, causal and atomic principles in relation to the five elements.

**VAISHNAVA** One who worships Vishnu in the form of Rama, Krishna, Narayana etc.

**VIDYA** Knowledge.

**VIJNANA** Intuitive ability of mind; higher understanding

**VINYASA** Steady flow of connected yoga postures linked with breath work in a continuous movement. For example: sun salutation.

**VAYU** Wind, prana.

**VIVEKA** Reasoning and discerning mind; right knowledge or understanding.

**VRITTI** Circular movement of consciousness; mental and modifications described in raja yoga

**YAMAS** In the Yoga Sutras, Patanjali defined five yamas or ways to relate to others (moral conduct). They are nonviolence; truth and honesty; nonstealing; moderation; and nonpossessiveness.

**YANTRA** Visual form of mantra used for concentration and meditation

**YOGA** Derived from the Sanskrit word for "yoke" or "join together." Essentially, it means union. It is the science of uniting the individual soul with the cosmic spirit.

**YOGA NIDRA** Technique of yogic or psychic sleep which induces deep relaxation

**YOGI** Someone who practices yoga.

**YOGINI** A female yoga practitioner.

**1** SURYANAMASKAR Salutation to sun
. Surya: sun
. Namaskar: greetings or salutation

**2** HASTAPADA ASANA Hands to feet Pose
. Hasta: hand
. Pada: foot or leg.

**3** TADASANA Palm tree pose.
. Tada: palm tree

**4** VRIKSHASANA Tree Pose
. Vriksha: tree

**5** HANUMANASANA Hanuman is the Great Warrior in form of monkey who helped Lord Rama.

**6** GARUDASANA Garuda, the eagle is known as King of birds and vehicle of Lord Vishnu.

**7** VATAYANASANA Horse Pose
. Vatayana: King of horses

**8** NATARAJASANA Nata means dancer and Raja means King. Nataraja means King of dancers, a dynamic form of Lord Shiva.

**9** MURGASANA Chicken Pose
. Murga : Chicken

**10** EKA PADA ASANA One Leg Balance Pose
. Eka: one

. Pada: foot or leg

**11** UTTHIT IPREETPASCHIMOTTANASANA Reverse Standing Back Stretch Pose
. Uthita: Standing
. Vipareet: Reverse, Opposite
. Pascha: Back
. Tana: Stretch

**12** UTTHIT TRIVIKRAMASANA Standing split devoted to Lord Vishnu
. Trivikrma – One of the forms of Vishnu as a warrior

**13** HASTHA ASANA Hand Balance Pose

**14** RATHACHARIYA ASANA Chariot Riding Warrior Pose
. Ratha: Chariot
. Achariya: Master, One who holds

**15** PADOTTANASANA Wide Leg Open Stretch Pose

**16** UTHITA TRIKONASANA Standing Triangle Pose
. Tri: Three
. Kona: Angle
. Trikona: Triangle

**17** SUPTA-VAJRASANA Lying Thunderbolt Pose
. Supta: Lying

. Vajra: thunderbolt

**18 LAGHU VAJRASANA** Small Thunderbolt Pose
. Laghu: small, little, tiny, miniature

**19 SHASHANKASANA** Rabbit Pose
. Shashanka: Rabbit

**20 USTRASANA** Camel Pose
. Ustra: Camel

**21 KUNDALINIASANA** Dormant Energy Pose
. Kundalini: Dormant energy resting or stored at base of the spine, coiled in form of snake in mooladhara chakra.

**22 MANDUKA ASANA AND MUDRAS** Frog Pose or Gesture
. Manduka: frog
. Mudra: seal or gesture

**23 VAJRA VEERA ASANA** Hero Pose
. Veera: Hero, Warrior

**24 VAJRA VEERIYA ASANA** Heroic Pose
. Veeriya: Endurance or stamina at mental, physical, emotional and spiritual levels, bravery, strength

**25 JANUSIRASANA** Head to Thigh Pose
. Janu: Thigh
. Sirsa: Head

**26 PASCHIMOTTANASANA** Back's Forward fold Pose
. Paschim: West

**27 KURMASANA** Turtle or Tortoise Pose
. Kurma: Turtle or Tortoise

**28 NIRALAMB PASCHIMOTTANASANA OR VAJROLIMUDRA** Unsupported Back's forward stretch
. Vajrolimudra: Thunderbolt Gesture
. Niralamba: Unsupported

**29 ARDHA-BADDH-PADAM-PASCHIMOTTANASANA** Bonded Half Lotus Back's Forward Stretch Pose
. Ardha: Half
. Baddha: Bonded
. Padam: Lotus

**30 GOMUKHASANA** Cow Face Pose
. Go (Gau): Cow
. Mukha: Face

**31 BHAIRAVASANA** Bhairava is a form of Lord Shiva worshipped in Tantra Yoga.

**32 DWIPADSHIRASANA** Both Feet to Head Pose
. Dwi: two

**33 KALBHAIRAVASANA** Fierce Bhairava Pose (this is another form of Lord Shiva, using his fierce form to kill the demons)

**34 BRAHMCHARYASANA** Celibacy Pose
. Brahmachariya: Celibacy

**35 ASTAVAKRASANA** Eight Angle

Pose
. Asta eight
. Vakra: angle, twist, turn
**36 AAKARN DHANURASANA** Bow To Ear Pose
. AAkarna: To the ear
. Karna: Ear
. Dhanura: Bow
**37 GARBHASANA** Womb Pose
. Garbha: Womb
**38 STAMBHAM ASANA** Pillar Pose
. Stambham: Piller
**39 BADDHA KONA ASANA** Bounded Feet Angle Pose
. Baddha: Bounded
**40 PRATIPAHALASANA** Reverse Plough Pose
. Pratipa: reverse
. Hala: plough
**41 YOGAMUDRASANA** Yoga Gesture Pose
. Yoga: Union
**42 PARVATASANA** Mountain Pose
. Parvata: Mountain
**43 RAJKAPOTASANA** Royal Pigeon Pose
. Raj: king, royal
. Kapota: Pigeon
**44 GUPTPADMASANA** Hidden or Secret Lotus Pose
. Gupta: secret, hidden
**45 KUKUTTASANA** Cockerel Pose
. Kukuta: Cockerel

**46 ARDHA MATSYENDRASANA** Half Matsendra: Asana.
**47 MATSYENDRASANA** Matsendra Natha is one of the well known master of Hatha Yoga and he taught that press your organs against your organs to awaken the dormant energies for spiritual awakening. Hence this group of asanas are named
**48 MARICHAYA ASANA** Pose Dedicated to Sage Marichi
**49 TITIBHASANA** Firefly Pose
. Titibha: Firefly
**50 DHANURASANA** Bow Pose
**51 BHUJANGASANA** Cobra Pose
. Bhujanga: Cobra
. Bhujangini: Female serpent
. Naga: King Cobra
**52 SHALBHASANA** Locust Pose
. Shalbha: Locust
**53 VIPREETPASCHIMOTTASANA** Reverse or Inverted Back's Stretch
**54 SARVANGASANA** Shoulder Stand Pose
. Sarva: All
. Anga: Body Parts, Organs
**55 HALASANA** Plough Pose
**56 VIPAREETA KARNI MUDRA** Reverse Action Gesture
. Karni: Action
**57 KARAN PEEDASANA** Knees to Ear Pose

. Karan: ear

. Peeda: knees

**58 SHIRSHASANA** Head Stand Pose

**59 KAPALASANA** Skull Pose

. Kapal: Skull

**60 NIRALAMBA SIRSHASANA** Unsupported Head Stand

. Niralamba: Unsupported

. Salamb: supported

**61 BAKASANA** Heron Pose

. Baka: heron

**62 BAKDHYANASANA** Heron Meditation Pose

. Dhyana: Meditation

**63 VRASHCHIKASANA** Scorpion Pose

. Vrishchika: Scorpion

**64 MAYURASANA** Peacock Pose

. Mayura: Peacock

**65 MAYURIASANA** Peahen Pose

. Mayuri: Peahen

**66 VASHISHTHATAPASYAASANA** Sage Vashistha Austerity Pose (Sage Vashistha used this pose to meditate )

. Vshishtha: A great sage and auther of yoga Vashistha and some other scriptures.

. Tapsya: Austerity

**67 CHAKRASANA** Wheel Pose

. Chakra: wheel, circle

**68 MATSAYASANA** Fish Pose

. Matsya: Fish

**69 YOGANIDRASANA** Yoga Sleep Pose

. Nidra: Conscious sleep

**70 SUPTA TRIKONASANA** Lying Triangle Pose

**71 SUPTATRIVIKRAMASANA** Lying leg split pose (this pose is also devoted to lord Vishnu as Trivikrama is one of his forms)

**72 NAVASANA** Boat Pose

. Nava: Boat

**73 SARVA ASANA** Whole Body Pose

. Sarva: All, Whole, Complete

**74 SETUBANDHASAN** Bounded Bridge Pose

. Setu: Bridge

. Bandha: Bounded

**75 PAVAN MUKTASANA** Wind Release Pose

. Pavan: wind

. Mukta: free, release

**76 SHAVASANA** Corpse Pose

. Shava: Corpse

**77 PADMASANA** Lotus Pose

**78 BADDHPADMASANA** Bounded Lotus Pose

**79 VAJRASANA** Thunderbolt Pose

**80 GORAKSHASANA** This pose is dedicated to Sage Gorksha, a great Nath Yogi.

**81 KANDPEEDASANA** Sole on Navel Pose

**82 SUKHASANA** Easy pose

. Sukha: easy, pleasant,

comfortable

**83** SWASTIKASANA Auspicious Pose
. Swastika: Hindu symbol of
Auspiciousness

**84** SIDDHASANA Perfect pose
. Siddha: perfect, mastered

Lightning Source UK Ltd.
Milton Keynes UK
UKOW04f2353050517
300584UK00005B/121/P